£5.95

D1637594

Palliative Care of the
Terminally Ill

Palliative Care of the Terminally Ill

J. F. HANRATTY

RADCLIFFE MEDICAL PRESS
OXFORD

© 1989 Radcliffe Medical Press Ltd
15 Kings Meadow, Ferry Hinksey Road, Oxford OX2 0DP

British Library Cataloguing in Publication Data

Hanratty, James
Palliative care of the terminally ill.
1. Terminally ill patients. care
I. Title
362.1'75

ISBN 1-870905-01-6

Printed and bound in Great Britain
Typeset by Advance Typesetting, Oxfordshire

Contents

Preface

During the last ten years, increasing numbers of doctors, nurses and students have visited St. Joseph's Hospice seeking information on hospice care. To assist with their teaching I produced three booklets and several papers to cover the whole range of problems encountered in terminal care. When Radcliffe Medical Press invited me to amalgamate these booklets and papers into one volume I took the opportunity to bring them up-to-date and to add several chapters, in particular one concerning Ethical Issues.

Most hospices are orientated towards the care of patients dying from cancer (which accounts for more than a quarter of all deaths in the U.K.), but the contents of this volume will apply to the care of patients dying from whatever cause.

Hospice care is synonymous with palliative care of the highest quality, but it is not the prerogative of hospices; it can be provided equally well in hospitals or in the patient's home.

The theme for this book can be summarized as 'Compassion with Competence'. We all have great compassion for our patients, but this needs to be supplemented by practical intervention to provide relief from their distress. Such intervention needs to be given with competence, and this requires some expertise and knowledge of what is available and appropriate, and the capability to apply it efficiently.

The first part of this book is concerned with the philosophy of terminal illness and should assist with the compassionate approach to patient care. The second part is orientated towards clinical care and is a guide for the control of distressing symptoms in the dying patient. It is hoped that this combination will assist doctors and nurses in their efforts to bring comfort to their patients in terminal illness and to the families.

In preparing the original booklets I had the assistance of various papers on terminal care written by Dr. R. Twycross of Sir Michael Sobell House, Oxford. 'The Management of Terminal Disease', edited by Dame Cicely Saunders, was also very helpful.

I would also like to acknowledge the many doctors, sisters and nurses who have been such wonderful colleagues during my ten years at St. Joseph's Hospice. I regret that they are too numerous to mention individually, but of particular help were Dr. Ray Corcoran and Dr. David Frampton, Sister Joan, Sister Marcella, Sister Catherine and Sister Jacqueline.

My thanks also to June Thompson for polishing up my writing, Gillian Nineham of Radcliffe Medical Press for suggesting this project, to Anita Hughes and Shirley Sasse for typing the script; and, last but by no means least, to my wife, Irene, for her unfailing support and constructive criticism.

DR. J. F. HANRATTY, O.B.E., K.S.G.,
Chairman, and formerly Medical Director
St. Joseph's Hospice, Hackney,
London E8

Philosophy of Terminal Illness

'Pray for me, O my friends; a visitant
Is knocking his dire summons at my door,
The like of whom, to scare me and to daunt,
Has never, never come to me before. . . .'

CARDINAL NEWMAN *The Dream of Gerontius*

Acceptance of the reality of death

The prospect of the awesome and inescapable finality of death fills most people with apprehension, fear or even stark terror. The remarkable advances of medicine in the last fifty years have reduced dramatically the numbers of those dying young or in the prime of life; death has largely been deferred to the old and very old and has become relatively remote. This is particularly evident in Western Society and has resulted in a death-denying attitude — a sort of naïvety whereby death is deliberately not thought of in the hope that by not thinking about it, it will just not happen. Increasing materialism and the diminution of religious interests do not always encourage the contemplation of one's ultimate fate. Life tends to be lived for the enjoyment of the moment; philosophising about the future being regarded as unrewarding.

Although most patients are aware of the nature of their illness, its history and remorseless progress, not all are prepared to talk about death. This reluctance must be respected by the carers whilst giving the patient every opportunity to discuss the subject. If the patient can be gently led to talk about the reality of death and express fears about it, much of the tension and anxiety felt may be alleviated.

The doctor and the dying patient

'To cure sometimes, to relieve often, to comfort always.'

Hippocrates

Despite the advances of modern medicine and expertise, some patients still die in utter misery, with unrelieved pain and with distressing symptoms inadequately controlled. It is particularly sad that this should happen when there are various therapies and medications readily available to give patients significant and in most cases complete relief from their suffering.

The management of terminal illness is all too often sadly mismanaged, although it is not an infrequent experience for the average doctor to be confronted with a dying patient.

This may be because during training, medical students are not adequately taught about symptom control in terminal illness; more likely it is because doctors by tradition and training are conditioned to do their utmost to cure a patient. This is right and laudable, but when they come to treat a dying patient and there is no prospect of a cure, their continued efforts may appear unrewarding.

They may feel that this failure to cure is a humiliating defeat and their kindly concern for the plight of the patient and family may lead to a feeling of helplessness. They may even utter that chilling phrase, so inept when coming from a doctor, 'there is nothing more I can do.' As a result there may be embarrassment when meeting the patient and the relatives and these meetings, which are both time consuming and emotionally demanding, may be short and reduced to the minimum compatible with essential treatment. Or they may be delegated to others. The patients and their families are quick to sense this withdrawal and their isolation and worries are inevitably made worse.

The converse may also occur when vigorous curative treatment continues to be given, which often involves extraordinary and sophisticated measures in a futile bid to keep the patient alive at all costs.

The usual result of this is to add to the distress of the patient and the family. It is never easy to determine exactly when to discontinue efforts to cure, and each patient poses unique problems. The final decision requires consultation with the family, medical and nursing colleagues, and if possible with the patient; indeed not infrequently it is the patient who will decide.

At St. Joseph's Hospice it is the practice to establish that the diagnosis is accurate and that death is not far distant.

A change of role and attitude is then required in the management of the illness by all those caring for the patient. There is nothing more to be done to *cure* the patient but there is an enormous amount to be done to *care* for the patient and to ensure that the remaining few weeks or months of their life are spent in comfort and free from mental and physical suffering. Dying, just the same as being born is a process requiring devoted and skilful medical and nursing care.

The nurse and the dying patient

The achievement of comfort and relaxation in the dying patient is very demanding on the professional skills of a nurse. Moreover, the nurse who is in frequent and intimate contact with the patient is in a special position to monitor treatment and report any new developments.

Nursing care is administered at a much slower pace than is usually possible in a busy general hospital where there are often conflicting pressures and priorities. The weak, vulnerable patient requires gentle unhurried handling. Extra time must be given to establish effective communication, to sit and listen, and to be observant of the non-verbal messages which indicate the particular needs or discomforts, and to be aware of the fears and loneliness of the dying patient.

A warm personality and an ability to convey this is a great asset in supporting the anxious patients and relatives. It is also important to be sensitive to the feelings of colleagues especially the young and inexperienced, and to help establish a close working relationship with other members of the caring team.

Nurses who are constantly working with dying patients need to have outside interests away from the working environment, in order to keep themselves fresh and to be able to give their best to patients.

Care of the dying patient

'I went to sleep; and now I am refreshed
A strange refreshment: for I feel in me
An inexpressive lightness, and a sense
Of freedom, as I were at length myself. . . .'

CARDINAL NEWMAN *The Dream of Gerontius*

Effective care of the patient during the last few weeks or months of life requires compassion, competence and constant attention to detail, with every aspect of the patient's condition being studied. The dying patient is still a living person and needs to be treated as such.

Symptoms causing distress need to be discovered, anticipated and then relieved by effective therapy. The threshold at which these symptoms, especially pain, causes distress varies widely. It is personal to each individual and the social, cultural, religious and ethnic background of the patients plays a part. It may however fluctuate from day to day — even hour to hour. It is for instance lowered if a patient is uncomfortable, tired, worried, afraid, angry or isolated; and conversely it is raised by sympathy, rest, understanding and a pleasing environment.

Patients therefore benefit by being given the opportunity for leisure activities compatible with their condition and interests. The loneliness of the bedridden or chair-bound patient needs to be combated with the help of the relatives and relaxed, unhurried staff. If those around the patient are always busy and in a hurry the patient will be reluctant to complain of discomfort and will refrain from communicating fears and anxieties. Devoted nursing in a bright, colourful environment is essential and the aim should be to give the dependent, vulnerable patient that sense of security, which comes from being surrounded with love and kindness.

No two patients are alike and each one needs individual study. It always helps if the purpose of therapy is explained beforehand and the patient's wishes about treatment should be respected.

When the patient is first seen a full medical and social history should be taken and a careful enquiry made about all symptoms (see Appendix 5). A close member of the family should also be interviewed if possible in order to discover any specific problems not mentioned by the patient and also to obtain a fuller knowledge of the patient's personal and domestic background.

An assessment of the patient's insight (knowledge of diagnosis and prognosis) and emotional state should also be made at the first interview.

Symptoms requiring attention in terminal illness are:

Pain	Fungating lesions
Dysphagia	Immobility
Sore mouth	Ascites
Micturition problems	Hiccough
Fistulae	Insomnia
Itching	Anorexia
Weakness	Dry mouth
Oedema	Diarrhoea
Cough	Discharge
Confusion	Skin trouble
Nausea and vomiting	Smell
Thirst	Paralysis
Constipation	Dyspnoea
Bleeding	Emotional problems
Pressure sores	Disfigurement

The control of these symptoms is discussed in detail in the second section of this book.

Communication in terminal illness

It is essential to keep the lines of communication open between the patient, doctor, staff and relatives. This can be done by regular ward meetings attended by the entire ward staff, social workers and chaplains, where discussion about patients and families who are posing problems can take place. Sometimes there may be concern about a patient who has particular needs or about relatives who are showing signs of strain and are in need of special support. The relevance of some therapeutic procedures may also need discussion.

Patients frequently present a different face to the various people caring for them and visiting them. They may, for instance, wish to present themselves as a 'good' patient to the doctor and make no complaints when the doctor enquires. But when the doctor has gone, they may be more forthcoming to the nurse or perhaps only to a particular person with whom they have developed some rapport. A complete picture of the patient will only emerge from a combination of the impressions of all those who are caring for them.

Even though the doctor has the responsibility of making the final decision, these meetings are mutually supportive and all present have the opportunity to express their feelings as regards the care of the patient and their families.

When patients and relatives need to have a chat, doctors and nurses should give generously of their time and never be in a hurry or indicate that they have a pressing engagement elsewhere. Time is one of the most valuable things we can give to our patients. Their time is running out and it is so important to enable them to make the most effective use of the time that is left.

As the patient's vital functions begin to disintegrate there is a constant change of symptoms, many of which may be anticipated by a knowledge of the pathological state of the patient.

All of these require constant study, and application of appropriate medical and nursing procedures to give comfort and to maintain the patient's personal dignity.

It is easy to assume that every symptom causing distress is from the cancer, whereas discomfort may arise from conditions other than the cancer — such as dyspepsia, haemorrhoids, arthritis or toothache and these should be relieved by appropriate specific treatment.

Patients are all too often given massive doses of tranquillizers or antidepressant drugs which render them dull, apathetic and drowsy. It is the policy at St. Joseph's Hospice to avoid the use of these drugs unless they are absolutely necessary, as the aim is to keep patients alert, lively, active and congenially occupied for as long as possible.

Depression in terminal illness may occur especially in patients who have a history of psychiatric illness. It may also affect patients whose terminal phase lasts for many months. These patients may need anti-depressants, but depression is not a very frequent feature of terminal illness. Sadness which is often confused with depression is an understandable emotion and is not helped by drugs at all. It is best treated by avoidance of isolation, interesting diversion and frequent opportunities for talking with the staff and supportive relatives, and, if appropriate, their pastors.

Whatever therapy is administered to the patient in terminal illness the doctor should ask himself or herself these questions:

Is this treatment really necessary for this patient at this time, i.e. is its purpose to give comfort and control distressing symptoms?

Has the treatment any undesirable side effects or complications? If so, can these be anticipated or minimized?

Is the treatment of sufficient importance to warrant a full explanation of its implications to the patient and/or relatives, giving them an opportunity to express an opinion with the option to accept or reject the treatment?

Communication with the patient

'I would have nothing but to speak with thee
for speaking's sake. I wish to hold with thee
Conscious communion; though I fain would know
A maze of things, were it but meet to ask. . . .'

CARDINAL NEWMAN *The Dream of Gerontius*

Communication with a dying patient is not easy − it is full of emotional hazards and very time consuming. It is not surprising that it is often avoided. Indeed not long ago it was regarded as tantamount to malpractice to divulge to a patient that their illness was terminal. All kinds of subterfuge were adopted to avoid the issue, as it was thought that no patient could accept such devastating knowledge. It was regarded as being both kindly and ethical to use any means, however devious, to avoid telling a patient the truth. Patients were too often fobbed off with facile reassurances.

Times have changed and modern society is much more enquiring and less prepared to take things on trust. However, when it comes to discussion of death there still persists that reluctance to give the patient any opportunity to come to terms with it. Doctors, nurses, families and friends still feel in many instances that they should shield the patient, and they unite in erecting a communication barrier. It is a flimsy barrier because so often they know the patient knows that the illness is terminal, and the patient knows that they know. This situation is perpetuated by constant avoidance of all reference to the patient's prospects. Conversation with the patient is kept on a superficial plane of banality and hollow cheerfulness.

People do not know what to say and are afraid of saying the wrong thing and their kindly sensitivity can lead to reticence. Little do they know that the majority of patients are eagerly awaiting the opportunity to talk about everything that is happening and in prospect. If this is denied them the consequent loneliness adds enormously to their emotional isolation.

Given a setting of easy and confident communication, seriously ill people make fewer complaints. If they are given the opportunity, they are only too willing to tell anyone prepared to listen what it is they fear, and if their anxiety can be settled then their pain threshold can be raised and a reduction of analgesic drugs often follows. Moreover, a spirit of frankness adds a new dimension to the relationship between doctor and patient.

There are some patients who prefer not to discuss such matters with the doctor — although virtually certain of the true prognosis. This reserve and the patient's unexpressed wish must be respected.

There are three guidelines in talking to patients:

1. Always tell the truth
2. Consider that patients, if they ask, have an absolute right to be told whatever they wish to know about their diagnosis and prognosis
3. Regard it equally as a right for patients not to have information which they are not seeking thrust upon them. It suffices therefore to give patients ample opportunity to signify their wishes

At the end of the first interview with the patient, an open and frank relationship can be initiated by the doctor saying 'Well, I have been asking all the questions so far, have you anything at all you want to ask me?' This gives the patient an early opportunity to achieve a rapport with the doctor and the response may be:

'What is the matter with me Doctor?'
'Will I get better?'
'I suppose it must be something serious'
'No thanks Doctor I've nothing special to ask'

The last response does not mean that on a later occasion another initiative from the doctor will receive the same response. It means that the patient at that time is not prepared to risk putting anxieties into words. Further opportunities should be given to the patient from time to time and once rapport is established the patient is much more likely to be responsive.

The doctor should always answer truthfully but instead of giving the truth harshly or unadorned it is better when answering the questions to turn them around and reply for instance, 'You have asked me that but before I answer, could you tell me what you yourself think about your condition?' It is often helpful at this stage to take the patient through the history of the illness step by step. Patients are usually well aware of the significance of certain symptoms, for example coughing or vomiting of blood, loss of weight, followed by a battery of tests, operations, radiotherapy and continuing ill-health. In this way most patients are able to work it out for themselves. The doctor should explain in simple, non-technical terms the nature of the illness and the prognosis.

It is impossible to soften the impact of bad news. However it is important to let the patient determine the pace of the discussion. Perception of the implications takes time and the patient's response may be very slow; it should be awaited quietly and peacefully.

'How long have I got?' is a frequent question and is difficult to answer accurately. It is very unwise for the doctor to give a fixed time, e.g. three months, six months etc. These estimates may occasionally be correct but more often they prove to have been wildly inaccurate, to the embarrassment, and sometimes the distress, of all concerned.

It is kinder therefore to err on the optimistic side when giving a prognosis. Temporary remissions may occur, and even complete regressions, though very rare, are not unknown. A mention of these, emphasizing their rarity, gives the patient that small grain of hope.

Hope indeed is relative to the circumstances. The big hope of course is for a complete cure and restoration to normal good health. Such hope is unrealistic and the patient knows this. There are however many little hopes and these can achieve great importance in the patient's day to day life, for example, hope for a family visit, hope to live long enough for a family celebration such as a birthday or anniversary or hope for a weekend at home.

Once the patient has achieved insight into the diagnosis and prognosis there follows a series of supplementary questions to be answered and anxieties to be resolved. The patient may not be able to comprehend everything on the first occasion and frequent contacts afterwards are essential. Non-verbal communications assist the development of a harmonious relationship − sitting down beside the patient, showing no indication of being in a hurry and giving full attention to everything discussed. Patients with terminal illness often feel the need for tangible contact with those caring for them, and shaking and holding hands gives physical expression to the personal relationship. It is not necessary for there to be constant conversation − sitting quietly in silence is immensely supportive.

After talking to a patient, a glance back after leaving the bedside is most instructive, as the patient's facial expression at that moment gives an uninhibited indication of their emotional state. A worried, frightened, anxious expression necessitates a return to the bedside as a patient in that state should not be left alone.

Case History

Mrs R. a frail but alert old lady in her early seventies, was admitted with a diagnosis of inoperable carcinoma of stomach. She had suffered for many years from severe rheumatoid arthritis for which she had been given a series of drugs−some of which have now been withdrawn due to their toxicity. Severe dyspepsia had led to her having a barium meal and the radiologist had reported this as showing a large, craggy ulcer in the lesser curvature typical of a malignant gastric ulcer. As there was a clinical suspicion of liver irregularity, and she was too frail to be subjected to surgery, no further investigations — not even endoscopy were performed. As she lived alone she was referred to the Hospice for terminal care. She had already been told that she was suffering from a cancer and had accepted this with resignation.

On admission she was vomiting, nauseated and had intermittent epigastric pain, but no induration was found. She was treated with ranitidine 150 mg bd and she was also given Nystan oral suspension for thrush. With supportive nursing and suitable nutrition her condition began to improve, she gained weight and the dyspepsia cleared. In view of her continual improvement over the following few months she was referred for re-investigations. A repeat barium meal was reported as normal and there was no sign of any malignancy. We had the pleasant task of informing her that she was free from cancer and after arranging for community support she was eventually discharged home.

While we do not wish to subject patients to a battery of investigations, some of which could be unpleasant, in order to confirm the diagnosis, this case illustrates the pitfalls in accepting a diagnosis from inadequate investigations.

Case history

Mr. L. had developed cancer of the nose — a most unpleasant and distressing form of malignancy. In his case it had resisted all attempts at curative treatment and on admission the large fungating tumour had destroyed the central part of his face causing gross distortion and disfigurement and giving the appearance of a gargoyle. A man of sensitivity he was embarrassed and withdrawn and wished to be isolated, but we soon found that behind this revolting "mask" there was a person of high intellect with a sense of humour and a gentle nature. Once we had got used to his thick speech caused by the cancer, conversation was relaxed and enjoyable and it was easy to forget that he had this disease, when relating to the person behind it. Indeed people were often queueing up to talk to him.

Treatment with antibiotics, including metronidazole for the foul-smelling anaerobic infection, Nystan for thrush, morphine and carbamazepine for the pain, made him much more comfortable, and when steroids were added there was significant reduction of the size of the tumour.

His history was interesting. He and his mother and sister were in a prison camp in Poland during the war. His mother and sister disappeared, but he was spared as he was only twelve years old. Eventually he came to London and became apprenticed as a watch repairer. Later he had a business of his own and married — there were no children. Sadly his wife died and he was left with no known relatives, but he was engrossed in his work and had many intellectual interests. After several months he was happily settled in the Hospice with the cancer quiescent. One day he was visited by some "friends" and following their visit his whole demeanour changed—depressed and withdrawn. Apparently these "friends" had said "Oh dear! You must have led a wicked life for God to have punished you in this dreadful way". Utterly distraught he told them that he had led an average sort of life and never thought of himself as wicked. From being content and indeed cheerful this visit had a destructive effect on his morale and he became despondent and withdrawn. "There must be something in what they said", was his comment. Although he responded to our efforts he was never able to regain his previous cheerful attitude. He died in his sleep a few months later.

This case history illustrates the damage that thoughtless remarks can cause to patients in terminal illness.

The reactions and fears of the dying patient

'Now that the hour is come my fear is fled;
And at this balance of my destiny,
Now close upon me, I can forward look
With a serenest joy.'

CARDINAL NEWMAN *The Dream of Gerontius*

Once a patient realizes that death is not too far distant it is essential to give ample time and opportunity for discussing the implications of this realization. Depending on the patient's religion and expressed wishes, the ministrations of a spiritual adviser should be arranged. Even if religious interests have lapsed, a renewal at this time can bring comfort and peace. A legal adviser may also be necessary to provide for an orderly disposition of material assets, and a social worker to help with domestic affairs.

Complete insight does not necessarily imply complete acceptance. Some patients do accept the knowledge of their impending death with quiet resignation and complete placidity. Others however, may have a kaleidoscope of changing emotions and it is important for those caring for the patient to be prepared for these emotions.

Denial

This may follow any temporary improvement. The patient rejects thoughts of dying and erects a mental barrier of denial. There may be talk about the future in unrealistic terms, but it is better not to argue as the denial is that patient's way of coping.

Anger

This may be expressed by constant grumbling and complaining, by spiteful aggressive behaviour and may be directed at anyone − family or staff. Patients showing real anger tend to be regarded as 'awkward people' and may become isolated. Staff and relatives find them difficult to deal with, and not relishing having to accept the patient's anger with tolerance, close and frequent contacts are avoided. The only effective way to help is to grasp the nettle of anger by encouraging an outpouring of emotion from the patient, and to kill that anger by demonstrating kindliness and love at all times by all who are in contact with the patient.

Guilt

A patient may accept approaching death as a just punishment for past misdeeds but may then feel that such a punishment is excessively harsh.

Blaming

Seeking a scapegoat may lead to unfair blaming which is often directed towards those who have done most for the patient, such as the family or doctors and nurses. Sometimes previous working conditions or even hospital investigations and surgery are blamed. Patients and their families may become quite obsessed about blaming and may even consider litigation. A full, frank and detailed explanation in simple terms is the most effective way of defusing the situation.

Sadness

This occurs when contemplating the loss of everything one has worked for; loss of family contacts and friends.

Depression

This is a less common reaction. It is more likely to occur in patients with a history of psychiatric instability and frequently responds to treatment with anti-depressants.

The patient's mood ranges through these emotions, oscillating from one to another, and often varying from day to day; with hope intervening. The emotions of the relatives often follow a similar pattern.

Once the reality of impending death is accepted various attitudes towards death may develop:

Death as a friend

This applies particularly to those with faith in a god. They may be able to face death with equanimity, as a homecoming and as a release from the tribulations of this world. There are however those who have no belief in any existence beyond this life and some of these may be capable of achieving an inner peace too. Others who regard death as a friend are those who feel that they have obtained what they could out of their lives and are now able to face death with fatalistic acceptance.

Death as an enemy

This affects those for whom the prospect of forced separation from all that is familiar, and from loving and intimate relationships leads to a feeling of utter desolation and loneliness. They become angry, bewildered and terrified and need constant support from the whole caring team.

Death as a challenge

This is similar to when the alarm is sounded for action stations in wartime. There is the prospect that something unknown is going to happen very soon and the ultimate outcome is uncertain. The feeling of apprehension is compounded with a determination to do one's duty with dignity − not to let oneself or others down, and to accept with resignation whatever may be the outcome.

Death the indignity

The fear of many is the prospect of pain unrelieved, the embarrassment of incontinence, the frustration of immobility and the dread of irrationality. The patient should be given ample time to express these fears, and needs to have confident reassurance of constant caring support.

Most people however do not formulate their feelings so rigidly. Equanimity may be sought by discussing these fears with a member of the caring team, with a relative, sympathetic friend or with a spiritual adviser. A patient should be encouraged to look for some goal of pleasure and enjoyment in each day:

> A visit from a friend today
> I went out into the garden today
> My favourite football team won today

Sometimes it helps to keep a diary recording each day's pleasures.

Many patients sitting quietly and thinking need some guidance and it helps to give them some themes for meditation:

> What have I done with my life?
> What achievement(s) can I look back on with satisfaction?
> Is there anything I really wish to do now before I become weaker?
> Whom do I really love and cherish?
> Who really loves and cherishes me?
> What does death mean to me?

For those who have a religious faith − prayer and contemplation, and arranging meetings with their religious pastors can assist in achieving spiritual peace and tranquillity.

A patient should be encouraged to be as busy as possible with enjoyable activities: reflecting on happy memories − holidays, family celebrations or achievements; browsing through a family photograph album; meditating on religious or spiritual themes. The consolation and comfort patients obtain will depend largely on the religious, cultural, social and ethnic influences in their lives.

The objective is for patients to 'live' until they die and not merely to exist.

Communication with the relatives

> 'What is termed the 'agony of death'
> concerns the watcher by the bedside
> rather than the one who is the subject of pity.'
>
> SIR FREDERICK TREVES

From the time the patient is admitted the close co-operation of the family should be sought as an essential contribution to the totality of care. The contact should continue throughout the illness to the death of the patient and extend through the bereavement for as long as it is needed. This may be for months or occasionally years.

The interview with the relatives at the time of admission, when salient information concerning the patient is obtained, also gives an opportunity to develop a friendly association. Frequent contact afterwards should be encouraged and can be facilitated by having flexible visiting times. The patient's illness often incurs family, financial or domestic difficulties, and the help of a knowledgeable and sympathetic social worker may bring considerable comfort to the often confused and frightened family.

Sometimes the family have a sense of guilt because the patient can no longer be kept at home. Often there have been prolonged and heroic efforts to continue the home care, and the relatives are greatly relieved to be reassured that the time has now come when in-patient care is essential.

Many relatives obtain much needed comfort by being allowed and encouraged, under guidance, to perform or assist with some parts of the nursing care. They can give practical and often very useful assistance, which is much appreciated by the patient and staff.

It is sometimes helpful to give relatives a few guidelines on visiting. Too many people should not visit at the same time, and there is no need for constant talk − especially the sort of talking which requires a response from the patient.

Sitting quietly, holding the patient's hand and enjoying the contact in silence, may seem strange at first but, once achieved, visits made in this way give great mutual comfort.

The understandable protectiveness of the relatives may extend to their desire to shield the patient from all knowledge of the diagnosis and prognosis. 'You won't tell will you doctor?' It is necessary at an early stage to point out that it is the patient who should decide, but at the same time, the relatives should be reassured that any discussion with the patient will be conducted in a gentle, soothing and supportive manner, and they will be kept fully informed.

Frequently the doctor and nurse are able to act as catalysts between patient and relative to achieve an openness, and ability to discuss the implications of the terminal illness. The consequent release of tension is a great comfort to everyone.

> 'It is incredible how much happiness
> even how much gaiety, we sometimes
> had together after all hope of recovery
> was gone. How long, how tranquilly,
> how nourishingly, we talked together
> that last night!'
>
> C. S. LEWIS *A Grief Observed*

Bereavement

> 'No one ever told me that grief felt so like fear.
> I am not afraid, but the sensation is like being afraid.
> The same fluttering in the stomach, the same restlessness . . .'
>
> C. S. LEWIS *A Grief Observed*

The general demeanour of those visiting the dying patient during the last few weeks should be observed discreetly by the caring staff. This will give some indication of those who are likely to need some further support during bereavement. The social worker should be alerted and briefed and follow-up visits made. These visits may have to continue over months or even years depending on the amount of support which is found to be necessary.

The death of a loved one inflicts grievous pain on those who were near and dear, and the pain is none the less, even if the death came as no surprise. The initial reaction is a feeling of numbness, disbelief, and even a denial that this can really have happened.

After the first few days of shock there develops an awareness of the reality of the death, and subsequent grief may take differing and fluctuating forms.

Anger

This is very frequent with a desire to throw things about and an impatience and irritability with everyone, even with those who are doing their best to help.

Guilt

This involves a recapitulation of the events leading up to the death, and an analysis of these events. 'If only I had done so and so this would not have happened.' Self-castigation leads to the agony of remorse. These thoughts can easily lead on to blaming others, 'If only *they* had done so and so, this would not have happened.' The sad thing about this train of thought is that very often those who have done the most to help, such as members of the family, doctors and nurses, are deeply hurt by this 'blaming'.

Disorganisation

This often follows due to lack of interest and unwillingness to apply the mind to the mundane requirements of day to day life.

Isolation

A withdrawal from social contacts may be due to a feeling of embarrassment at causing others to feel uncomfortable should an attack of uncontrollable weeping occur. There is also the awkwardness of conversation even with close friends; an artificiality and superficiality when people constantly try to avoid any reference to the one subject that is uppermost in everyone's mind. The sensation of being an object of pity when appearing in public makes many people prefer to isolate themselves from friends and neighbours. Another cause of isolation is that they just cannot be bothered to make the effort to go out and about.

There is a significant increase in the morbidity and mortality of widows and widowers during the first year of bereavement as compared with those of similar age and background who have not been bereaved. This may well be due to self-neglect and isolation, or a diminished will to overcome adversity.

The care of the bereaved

'Blessed are they that mourn: for they shall be comforted.'

Matthew 5:4

Anticipatory care may often diminish the intensity of subsequent grief, by giving every possible support to those visiting the dying patient; by ensuring that the patient's distressing symptoms are effectively controlled; and by having an affectionate relationship with the patient and the family. The bereaved will then be able to look back and re-live those stressful weeks with some satisfaction.

'After all the death was so peaceful'

'Everything possible was done'

The funeral is not the grand finale. The next day is normal for others, but not for the bereaved and it is difficult to adjust to life as a half of a Mr. and Mrs., or without a partner, parent, child or other close relative or friend. They have lost a companion, a sexual partner, a mother/father of children and a confidante.

The most effective way to help the bereaved is to achieve a relaxed relationship whereby it becomes easy to talk freely about the one who has died. Let the bereaved person talk, and talk uninhibitedly about anything and everything connected with the one who has died. Dwelling on family memories, looking at old photographs, and having someone available to listen sympathetically are some of the ways of obtaining comfort and consolation. It is important to avoid platitudes such as: 'Time will cure', 'Go away for a holiday to help you forget', 'Don't keep dwelling on it all'. These are meaningless and can be hurtful.

Grief is the price paid for love and if it could all be forgotten so easily by the passage of time, by having a holiday, by not dwelling on it, that loving relationship must indeed have been fragile and without substance. The passage of time helps to assuage the grief but will never eradicate it; the scar will always remain.

The purpose then, in caring for the bereaved, should be to achieve re-integration rather than substitution.

The use of drugs such as tranquillizers and anti-depressants conspicuously fails to give more than ephemeral comfort to the bereaved. Occasionally a pathological depression may occur which necessitates psychiatric treatment and the use of anti-depressant drugs. Apart from these cases drugs should be prescribed very sparingly in the treatment of the bereaved − perhaps the occasional night sedative in the first few weeks and nothing further. Many people become drug dependent after drugs have been prescribed to treat bereavement.

Much help may be given to the bereaved by putting them in touch with others in a similar situation. Cruse, The Society of Compassionate Friends and the Samaritans can provide useful support (see Appendix 2). Financial advice may also be necessary and the social worker should be able to advise on benefits and welfare rights. Further help can also be obtained from organisations such as Age Concern, One Parent Families and Child Poverty Action Group (see Appendix 2).

When appropriate the bereaved should be encouraged to have recourse to their religious faith and seek the guidance of their pastor and the companionship of fellow members of that faith. It may be months, even years, before the bereaved person succeeds in becoming effectively adjusted to everyday life without the support of the one who has died.

> To everything there is a season,
> and a time to every purpose under the heaven:
> A time to be born, and a time to die . . .
> A time to mourn . . .
> A time for peace . . .
>
> Ecclesiastes 3:1−8

Financial problems may add to the burden for many bereaved people, especially if the partner has been chronically sick for some time and has not been able to work. Often people are reluctant to disclose these problems however, and gentle probing may be necessary to find out whether the family has sufficient income to pay for the funeral costs, and to live on afterwards.

The hospice social worker, local social services department, or the social security office should be able to advise on welfare benefits available. Welfare rights offices, or Citizens Advice Bureaux are also able to help when there are legal or financial difficulties.

One very useful leaflet, issued by the Department of Social Security is D49 − *What to do after a death*. This includes practical information on arranging a funeral, what to do with property and possessions and where to get help.

Supplies can be obtained from the local social security office or from the address in Appendix 2.

Home care

> 'Be it ever so humble, there's no place like home.'
> J. H. PAYNE (1792)

Most people if asked where they would prefer to be for their final illness would opt for their own home, provided that essential care would be available. Understandably, patients are more relaxed and more content when they are in the familiar surroundings of their own home and in the presence of their own loving family. About forty or fifty years ago most patients (about two thirds) did remain at home for their final illness. Now it is the converse and over two thirds of deaths occur away from home − in hospitals, hospices or residential nursing homes.

When it is apparent that a patient is nearing the terminal stage of a progressive, incurable illness, a meeting of all interested parties should be held − patient, family, doctor and nurse − to discuss future management and plans. Certain questions require answers.

What are the patient's wishes?

What are the carer's/carers' wishes?

Is the home suitable?

Are there the necessary amenities, e.g. heating, bath, lavatory, and are these conveniently accessible?

Should the patient be moved to another room?

Who is available to provide the care at home and are they willing, available and capable (if there are several available, make out a rota)?

Are there good communications such as a telephone? Otherwise what are the plans for obtaining assistance?

Secure the help of community services (see Caring for the carers below)

Are the general practitioner and nursing services able to carry the burden of frequent and sometimes lengthy visits?

What other support, e.g. Macmillan nurses or hospice home care services are available?

Make advance plans on what to do should home care support break down, or patient and/or carers change their minds and prefer in-patient care.

Is there an adjacent hospice? In any case contact the nearest hospice to obtain advice on specific problems.

While transfer to in-patient care may become necessary and be the correct decision, it is always a traumatic experience if this is deferred until the last moment when the patient is 'in extremis' and may die on the journey, or shortly after in-patient transfer. Perhaps the most important aspect of home care is continuity of care by the same team of doctors and nurses. Emergency visits from total strangers are a poor substitute.

The carers and patient should understand clearly what medication is being given and what it is for. A chart listing all medication with times of dosage should be left in the house. Medical and/or nursing notes left in the house should be simple and clear to explain to colleagues so that someone unfamiliar with the patient will be able to provide appropriate treatment. Carers must always be kept fully informed about treatment, and ample time should be given to answer their queries and give them the support they need.

Always visit when the patient dies. The patient is beyond our care but the bereavement support for the family is just beginning. It is important to remember that in home care the roles are reversed from in-patient care. Doctors and nurses are the visitors; patient and family the hosts. Appropriate courtesies should always be observed.

Caring for the carers

This is a rough translation of the Latin phrase, 'Quis custodet ipsos custodes', which indicates that it is an age-old problem; indeed it is a problem as old as human life itself. Sadly, its importance is still frequently unrecognized.

The carer at home

Since the last war there have been fundamental changes in our Western Society resulting in smaller families, dispersed families, more women working outside the home and different social attitudes. An illness at home can have serious consequences for the carer who may try to continue with an outside job for fear of losing it. Many homes are run on a financial 'knife-edge' and loss of income is disastrous.

The carer at home is usually a woman − mother, daughter, or an in-law, and occasionally no relation at all, e.g. a kindly landlady or neighbour. The professional carers such as doctors, nurses, social workers, however devoted, are just short-term visitors to the home, and the continuing strain of coping with a seriously ill person inevitably rests with the resident carer, often with no respite.

The effect of the unrelenting responsibility will soon lead to various forms of tension. The carer will feel isolated, unable to enjoy normal social activities and have a diminished quality of life. Loss of sleep and ordinary relaxation will affect general health and eventually lead to reduced sympathy towards the patient and consequent feelings of guilt. The professional carers must be aware of these incipient problems and anticipate them by providing appropriate support right from the beginning such as:

- reassurance that someone will always be available should anxieties arise, for example where is the nearest telephone if there is none in the home?
- volunteer support from local community, for example church, neighbours, etc.
- arranging a night sitter, Marie Curie nurse, Meals on Wheels, laundry service
- periodic attendance at a Day Centre if there is one available and if the patient's condition permits
- respite admissions to local hospice or hospital
- ensuring that all statutory supplementary payments are being received
- trying to arrange that professional care is given by the same people. It is upsetting if total strangers arrive knowing nothing about the circumstances.

The carer in hospice or hospital

If patient care is provided by a team consisting of doctors, nurses, paramedical and social workers, the team should have regular meetings to discuss the care of patients and their families. Patients frequently show a different face to different members of the team, being quiet and reserved to some and chatting freely and uninhibitedly to others. At these meetings all present should be free to express their views about all aspects of patient and family care, and also their own personal attitudes. The meetings also provide mutual support and an opportunity to share with colleagues the stressful aspects of the work.

Other guidelines for staff support

There should be easy and informal access to senior members of the team, for example ward sisters and doctors who should be prepared to give ample time for discussion of problems and tensions.

Staff should be carefully observed by seniors for early signs of strain. Effective training should be provided so that staff are fully aware of the philosophy of palliative care and recreation and leisure activities encouraged.

Careful selection of staff is essential. This work is not suitable for those who have had a recent bereavement or a history of emotional instability.

Ethical issues in terminal illness

Communication

This is dealt with at length in previous chapters. It cannot however be over-emphasized that open and honest communication on all sides is paramount in achieving trust in terminal care. The relationship between doctors, nurses, patient and family is based on trust, it is fostered by friendliness and it is destroyed by deceit or suspicion; and once destroyed it can never be regained.

Prognosis is an inexact art and the short answer should always be 'I don't know', although it will be necessary to qualify this and discuss the patient's condition in more detail. Assessments in terms of days, weeks or months should be avoided. What is quite reprehensible is to tailor the prognosis in over-optimistic terms to suit and please the patient, while giving a completely different prognosis to others.

Refusal of treatment

It is a patient's right to accept or refuse treatment. It is however essential that the patient should realize the implications so that an informed decision can be made. A full, detailed and impartial explanation should be given; ample time for discussion and, if necessary, further professional opinion should be made available.

Some patients understandably reject chemotherapy or surgery for fear of unpleasant complications. The pros and cons should be set out clearly. A refusal is easier to accept if it is treatment unlikely to produce a cure, or will just provide temporary amelioration at the expense of much discomfort. Patients, because of their illness are essentially vulnerable and should not be pressurized to make a decision which conflicts with their inclinations. However, what is harder for the carers to accept is when a patient refuses treatment which will certainly give comfort and relieve distress, for example, a patient who refuses to have morphine for severe pain. Nevertheless, such a refusal must be accepted if that is the patient's firm and informed decision. The acceptance by the carers of such a decision must be complete and the patient must not be treated with discourtesy for going against the carers' advice. The care staff should not become sulky. Refusal of treatment may be by a patient who is mentally confused or paranoid. Here persuasion may be used and often succeeds. It is quite wrong to disguise drugs and give them surreptitiously, for example in their food or drink. If however a patient has a florid psychosis where sedation is vital, it is then justifiable to administer a drug against the patient's wishes as this is for the patient's own safety.

Fringe or unorthodox treatment

It is understandable when patients are suffering from a progressive, incurable illness, which has not responded to orthodox medicine, that they should seek treatment from unorthodox sources. Such treatment may be an anathema and offensive to the patient's doctors but, provided it is offered and given in good faith and is not likely to do any harm, for example certain types of diet or exercises, it must be accepted.

There are however 'fringe' treatments promulgated dishonestly and purely for monetary gain from vulnerable people. Patients and families should be dissuaded in very strong terms from submitting to the blandishments of charlatans.

Ordinary and extraordinary treatment

It is the fundamental duty of those caring for the patient to provide at all times what is termed ordinary treatment, and it is the patient's right to have, and to expect to be given such treatment. Ordinary treatment is that which is necessary to give comfort to the patient, for example the relief of distressing symptoms by appropriate medication and therapy; kindly, sympathetic nursing care, and assistance with natural functions and mobility; provision of, and assistance in taking, adequate nutrition and fluids.

Extraordinary treatment is an aggressive application of therapies over and above ordinary treatment and given in order to achieve a cure or prolongation of life; but at the same time is treatment which has inherent risks and complications. These need to be balanced against the chances of a successful or acceptable outcome.

Problems of decision arise because what is at one time ordinary treatment may at another time, and in the same patient, become extraordinary treatment. For example, the provision of adequate nutrition and fluids would become extraordinary treatment for the patient in semi-coma whose life is drawing to a close.

Whenever extraordinary treatment is contemplated, it should be preceded by full and frank discussions with everyone concerned — the patient, if this is possible, close relatives, and senior medical and nursing colleagues. There should be full documentation of all discussions and also of the treatment.

Examples of extraordinary treatment include: surgical by-pass for intestinal obstruction due to abdominal carcinomatosis; aggressive chemotherapy and life support resuscitation. Someone, and it is usually the doctor, has to make the final decision whether or not to give extraordinary treatment; but the patient's wishes if known should be paramount.

Ethical problems in ethnic groups

Communication

Language difficulties pose many problems especially if the patient and family come from an ethnic group with its own language. Every hospice needs to have pictures which can be used in obtaining information from the patient and the family while awaiting the services of an interpreter. It is essential to have a panel of interpreters from whom assistance may be obtained very rapidly. If an uncommon language is met, an approach to the appropriate Embassy will often be successful in obtaining someone knowledgeable in the language. The requirements of the care of patients in terminal illness involve close rapport with patient and family and if this has to be done through an interpreter it can be very time consuming and exhausting for everyone. Nevertheless it is absolutely essential that effective interpretation be achieved so that the patient and the family are fully cognisant of the patient's illness, prognosis, and treatment being given, and also to be able to answer questions and express anxieties and fears.

Occasionally the communication is complicated by an element of distrust which is based on fear, unfamiliarity, and lack of knowledge of the procedures of medical and nursing care in the U.K. This can require prolonged and careful discussion in order to eradicate the distrust and again can be extremely difficult if it has to be done through an interpreter, but nevertheless it must be done.

Cultural attitudes may cause problems. For example, there are some ethnic groups where women are not allowed to express any opinions for themselves and the men regard it as their duty to monitor every aspect of care including medical and nursing procedures. This attitude sometimes arouses antagonism in the female nursing staff who resent the fact that the women have been kept so subservient.

Non-acceptance of orthodox medical care

Frequently ethnic groups have been cared for by their ˎ
friends, some of whom may have no medical or nursinɓ
country. There may also be problems of diet which at timɛ.
indeed militate against orthodox medical care. Explanation is esɔ
full details of what is involved.

Non-acceptance of the philosophy of hospice care

The philosophy of hospice care as practised in the U.K. is that the time comes
in terminal illness when continued efforts to cure the patient are irrelevant and
inappropriate as the patient's condition has extended beyond the stage where
cure is possible. Continuing care therefore is concerned with relieving suffering
and controlling distressing symptoms as well as emotional support for the patient
and the family.

There are some ethnic groups who will not accept this philosophy and insist
that the patients are given the equivalent of intensive care right through to the
very end. Hospices are not equipped to provide this type of care and problems,
particularly in relation to the family, may result. It is therefore most important
to explain to the family the philosophy of hospice care at the very beginning in
order to avoid these misunderstandings.

Religious and cultural attitudes

The staff of the hospice must be at all times prepared to welcome, inform and,
in so far as it is possible, co-operate with the legitimate pastors of the patient
and family. 'Legitimate' pastors are occasionally well-meaning but interfering,
and sometimes aggressive friends or neighbours may present themselves as
representatives of the patients' and families' interests. It is therefore important
that pastors should be known as legitimate religious leaders.

The hospice must make itself aware of the religious and cultural attitudes of
various ethnic groups with regard to the practices adopted when the patient dies
and also with the procedures for the care of the body and its disposal.[1] The
hospice should have readily available as much information as possible on these
cultural and religious practices.

Disruption may occasionally be caused by these cultural and religious
procedures especially for other patients and their families, for example, ritual
wailing, and in this case a suitable side ward should be available for patient and
family.

[1] Caring for Dying People of Different Faiths, Rabbi Julia Neuberger

Euthanasia

The humanitarian and emotional reactions aroused in those observing someone severely disabled, diseased or dying are understandably distressing — particularly for the family. Not knowing what to do or what to say to alleviate apparent suffering leads to frustration and helplessness. The suffering in many cases is on the part of the beholder not the patient.

It is a dreadful indictment of our medical services that one of the main arguments in favour of euthanasia is that some people do die in physical and mental distress. However the patient should not have to be killed in order to stop distress. Patients in terminal illness, occasionally with the agreement of their family, may ask, either explicitly or by veiled hints, for an early end to their illness, i.e. they want the doctor to kill them.

This request should be regarded as a cry for help and it should not be brushed aside or ignored. It is easy to say 'That cannot be done, it is illegal' (which of course it is) and leave it at that. What is essential is to have long and detailed discussions with the patient to identify the problem (or problems) which prompted the request. The usual reason is fear or even terror of the process of dying which is anticipated as being accompanied by unrelieved physical distress such as pain or suffocation. These fears should be explored in depth and can be rapidly dissipated by establishing close rapport, gaining the patient's confidence, giving firm reassurance that symptoms will be relieved, and that someone known and trusted will always be available. Other reasons are loss of self esteem, a feeling that life is now useless and that they are a burden to everyone and emotional and spiritual desolation. It is always important to impress on patients that, despite the fact that their condition is such that they are constantly receiving, they are nevertheless unwittingly giving; giving of themselves and of their personalities. We the carers and their family are grateful to them for their presence and for the opportunity just to be with them.

Contact with the religious pastor, encouragement with recreational activities and enhancing personal appearance all help to bring comfort and tranquility and counteract the despair underlying the request for euthanasia. The confident reply to such requests is palliative care of the highest quality to enable patients to *live* until they die.

Nevertheless, there are those who with kindly intentions continue to campaign for voluntary euthanasia to be legalized. They do not realize that what they are seeking is veterinary medicine in preference to Hippocratic medicine. Moreover, the unique and inviolable quality of human life is a fundamental tenet of the Judaio-Christian religions. If euthanasia were to be legalized, some patients out of altruism might suggest it themselves: 'I don't want to be a nuisance'; 'I'm just spoiling their lives'. On the other hand knowing that euthanasia was permissible patients might begin to suspect their doctor's actions.

Inevitably the attitudes of doctors and nurses would harden, with a diminishing respect for the unique quality of human life. Indeed they would soon start to encourage patients to accept euthanasia (particularly those patients posing difficult medical and nursing problems). Doctors would find themselves conniving at assisted suicide; a socially dangerous and negative approach which confirms the patient's despair and denies all hope.

Euthanasia would be damaging and divisive to the family. Subsequent guilt reactions, accusations, recriminations and dissensions would have serious repercussions throughout the family.

A society accepting euthanasia would soon become a sick society itself. Once it was realized that when a human life became difficult to sustain and could be eliminated by euthanasia, this practice would be encouraged and in the long term even become mandatory.

After a year of deliberations a British Medical Association Working Party on Euthanasia reported in 1988. Its conclusion was that 'The Law should not be changed and the deliberate taking of a patient's life should remain a crime.'

Case history

In 1968, Mr. E., then aged 38, had a nocturnal fit, was taken to hospital, and after a stormy illness (encephalitis with bulbar palsy) ended with almost complete quadriplegia, dysphagia and aphasia. He had been a pilot officer in the R.A.F. and on demobilization was sales manager in an electronics firm, married with two children.

During the early stages, laborious communication was established with the help of his wife and an alphabet board — nodding his head when the correct letter was indicated. On admission to St. Joseph's Hospice in 1974 his quadriplegia was complete, apart from weak movements of his right index finger. He could nod his head and was still unable to speak, but his dysphagia was less troublesome. He had experienced periods of profound depression and frustration.

Gadgets were made to maximize his finger movement enabling him to touch type and thereby to communicate. Later he was able to paint with assistance with a palette. He is still at St. Joseph's and his disability is just as profound as when he was admitted, needing comprehensive nursing care and physiotherapy for his quadriplegia and medical care for occasional chest and urinary tract infections.

He has a very busy life, corresponding with numerous friends, has written a book 'The Long Road Back', goes home for most weekends, and with the help of family and friends has had holidays in Portugal and Switzerland. He has painted many very attractive pictures and is experimenting with glass engraving.

In the early days he was devastated at the prospect of life with such a major disability, but having got through that period with the help of his devoted wife and family, he is now enjoying a full, interesting and busy life. He is certainly glad that euthanasia was not available as he would have accepted it eagerly in the early days of his illness.

Control of distressing symptoms

Pain

Preamble

Pain in terminal illness, for example advanced cancer, can be classified in four main groups, all of which require specific attention:

Physical
Mental [anxiety, depression]
Social [isolation, embarrassment]
Spiritual [desolation]

This list can also be regarded from a different standpoint. If someone has overwhelming *physical* pain there are mental consequences such as inability to concentrate (such a patient will not wish to read or do a crossword); social consequences (the patient has no desire to talk and may just turn away 'go away and leave me alone'); spiritual consequences (a sense of despair and 'What have I done to deserve this'). Just as the pathological condition is destroying the patient physically so may it also as a consequence destroy the patient mentally, socially and spiritually.

Such unremitting pain is not like the acute ephemeral pain of a minor injury, nor does it have any protective or useful purpose. The priority therefore is to treat the physical pain rigorously and effectively.

Pain analysis

To establish the nature of the pain a full description should be obtained from the patient and from the family, paying particular attention to its onset, severity, location and character; and also its relationship to meals, movement, bowels, micturition and emotion.

Pain threshold

This is idiosyncratic and is determined by social, cultural, religious, familial and ethnic factors. It is also variable and may be lowered by fear, anger, isolation, loneliness, restlessness and depression. Conversely it may be raised by rest and adequate sleep, sympathy, diversion, congenial surroundings, confidence in the carers and good communication. The first line of attack on pain therefore is to do everything possible to raise the pain threshold.

Incidence of pain in advanced cancer

The general experience is that about 25% of patients have little or no pain, or such pain as they have is relieved by mild analgesics. This means that about 75% have pain requiring stronger analgesia, i.e. opiates, at some time in their final illness.

In a survey at St. Joseph's Hospice to find the proportion of patients in severe pain, we took an arbitrary dose of 30 mg of oral morphine 4 hourly and found that 33% of our patients needed this level of dosage or more at some time. Effective pain control is therefore a major challenge for those caring for terminally ill patients.

Mild pain

This only needs mild analgesics. Aspirin is a safe and effective minor analgesic for most patients and it is included in the formulation of a large number of analgesic preparations, mostly in a combination with paracetamol and/or codeine. The main disadvantage of aspirin is its tendency to cause gastric irritation in some patients. To overcome this, many formulations have been devised, e.g. enteric coated, delayed release or combinations with antacids. Paracetamol does not have the disadvantage of gastric irritation but it may cause constipation. Codeine is a centrally acting narcotic with approximately one tenth the analgesic potency of morphine to which it is metabolized in the body. Dextropropoxyphene is a weak, synthetic narcotic similar to methadone. Some suitable mild analgesics include:

> Soluble aspirin, 300 mg − 2 four hourly
> Co-codamol − 2 four hourly
> Co-proxamol − 2 four hourly
> Paracetamol 500 mg − 1 or 2 four hourly
> Benoral [benorylate] suspension 10 mls bd
> Ponstan [mefenamic acid] 500 mg tds (may cause diarrhoea)
> DF 118 [dihydrocodeine] 30 mg − 2 tds (may cause constipation)

Severe pain

As soon as it is apparent that these or similar mild analgesics are no longer effective there should be no hesitation in using the strong opiates.

Unfortunately these drugs are often withheld for fear of drowsiness, addiction or respiratory depression. Drowsiness, if it does occur, soon wears off.

Addiction is irrelevant in terminal illness, and in any case it is the general experience that when opiate drugs are given regularly under strict control of dosage and administration and for the control of specific symptoms, addiction does not occur. Respiratory depression is rarely a problem and is insignificant in comparison with the overriding benefit patients receive by having effective pain control.

Guidelines for use of opiate drugs

These should be given in adequate strength earlier rather than later in the illness. Once the correct dose has been ascertained they should be administered regularly and given in a form to ensure absorption. The dose should be monitored frequently, and side effects such as nausea and especially constipation, controlled.

It is unwise to administer opiates mixed with other drugs as in a 'strong analgesic mixture' or 'Brompton Cocktail'. This method allows for no flexibility and if the dose needs to be increased, the dose of the adjuvant drugs is also increased, risking undesirable side effects. Cocaine, which was a constituent of 'Brompton Cocktail', is no longer used as it has no beneficial effect.

Oral administration of opiates

Morphine sulphate is the drug of choice for oral administration. Diamorphine (heroin) is preferred by some doctors but there is not much to choose between the two so long as it is remembered that they are not equipotent. Diamorphine is a 'pro-drug' as it is rapidly de-acetylated *in vivo* to morphine, and it is as morphine that it exerts its analgesic effect. Diamorphine is also ten times more soluble than morphine, i.e. 1 g morphine needs 20 ml of water for solution and 1 g diamorphine needs 2 ml of water for solution. However, diamorphine when dispensed as a mixture, is less stable than morphine and should be used within ten days. The approximate oral equivalence of the two drugs is that diamorphine is 1.5 times more potent than morphine, i.e. 10 mg diamorphine equals 15 mg morphine.

Morphine sulphate is also available in slow release form [MST Continus] in doses of 10 mg [brown tablet], 30 mg [purple tablet], 60 mg [orange tablet] and 100 mg [grey tablet]. These are released slowly from the matrix over twelve hours and are administered twice daily.

Other opiate drugs with morphine equivalence are:

Pethidine [meperidine] 100 mg = 10 mg morphine
Dilaudid [hydromorphone] 1 mg = 6 mg morphine
Physeptone [methadone] 5 mg = 7.5 mg morphine
Palfium [dextromoramide] 5 mg = 15 mg morphine

Dromoran [levorphanol] 1.5 mg = 8 mg morphine
Omnopon [papaveretum] 5 mg = 5 mg morphine
Narphen [phenazocine] 5 mg = 15 mg morphine [may also be
given sublingually]
Diconal [dipipanone HCL 20 mg and cyclizine 30 mg] = 5 mg
morphine

Temgesic sublingual [buprenorphine HCL] 0.2 mg is a partial antagonist and should not be used at the same time as other opiates. It is occasionally of use as an intermediate analgesic before moving to regular opiate administration.

Palfium has too short a half life for routine use but it may be used as a supplement, for example, before some potentially painful procedures. Physeptone has a long half-life and a tendency to cumulation especially in the elderly, but it may help as a nocturnal supplement. Pethidine and Fortral [pentazocine] are unsuitable for the severe pain of terminal cancer as they are not potent enough and have a tendency to cause confusion.

Establishing the dosage of opiates

When commencing oral opiate medication, in a patient no longer experiencing pain relief from mild analgesics, the first prescription should be Rx morphine sulphate 5 mg, syrup or appropriate flavouring as required, chloroform water to 10 ml, dose − 10 ml every 4 hours. The dose of morphine has to be titrated against the patient's pain, and if there is breakthrough pain the next day, the dose is increased to 10 mg four hourly and thereafter in increments of 5 mg daily, until the patient is pain-free throughout the 24 hours; that is then the correct dose for that patient's pain at that time. After 20 mg 4 hourly, daily increments are 10 mg and after 100 mg 4 hourly, daily increments are 20 mg. It is much easier to establish the correct effective dose by using the morphine as a medicine but once the dose is established, transfer to slow release tablets [MST Continus] is easy, i.e. a patient who needs 20 mg morphine 4 hourly as a medicine is taking 120 mg morphine daily; this could then be given as an alternative in the form of MST Continus 60 mg bd.

Rectal administration of opiates

If oral medication is inappropriate, because of vomiting, dysphagia, weakness or suspected malabsorption, rectal administration may be considered. Provided there is no rectal pathology hindering insertion, or pelvic pathology affecting absorption, the result of rectal administration is almost as good as that of oral. Morphine suppositories are available in strengths of 15 mg, 30 mg and 60 mg and as with oral medication they must be given 4 hourly. Prolodone [oxycodone] suppositories are also available in a strength of 30 mg, equivalent to 15 mg morphine and only need to be given three times a day.

Parenteral administration of opiates

If oral or rectal administration are impossible, the opiate has to be given by injection. Diamorphine is clearly the drug of choice for injections as its greater solubility enables larger doses to be given in a smaller volume of fluid. Diamorphine is twice as potent as morphine − 5 mg diamorphine = 10 mg morphine when given by injection.

The potency by *injection* of both morphine and diamorphine is twice as much as when given *orally*. Accordingly, when transferring from oral to injection administration the dose should be halved.

Injections are given intramuscularly or subcutaneously. The intravenous route is never used.

If 4 hourly injections are required it is far better to use the Graseby syringe driver [MS 16]. If not available one may be borrowed from the local health department, hospice, hospital or the Lisa Sainsbury Foundation [see Appendix 2]. A 24 hour dose of the diamorphine [an anti-emetic may be added if necessary] is drawn into a 10 ml syringe which is fitted into the driver to which a cannula, with a butterfly needle, is attached. The setting is adjustable to deliver the contents of the syringe at a controlled rate, usually over 24 hours. The butterfly is inserted subcutaneously (usually in the suprascapular region), never into an oedematous region. Excellent and continuous pain control is achieved with this method and often with a smaller total dose of medication. The syringe is re-charged daily and it is wise to change the site of the needle every two or three days. Occasionally local indurations develop at the needle site but these are nearly always caused by phenothiazines which have been added to the diamorphine as anti-emetics.

A useful formula when changing from oral morphine to administration of diamorphine via the syringe driver is to divide the daily dose of morphine by three. This gives the daily dose of diamorphine, i.e. if a patient is receiving 20 mg of morphine 4 hourly the daily dose is 120 mg divided by three = 40 mg. Therefore the dose of diamorphine in the syringe driver is 40 mg daily.

Side effects of opiates

Nausea and vomiting are often initial reactions and wear off after a few days, enabling anti-emetics [if these have been given] to be reduced or withdrawn (see p. 38). Constipation is very common in patients taking opiates and laxatives should be prescribed routinely for all patients taking them. Once established constipation can be intractable and cause great distress (see p. 42). Sweating, dizziness, blurred vision and confusion occur occasionally, but they are usually transitory. For an opiate overdose, Narcan [naloxone] 0.4 mg by intravenous injection should be given.

Co-analgesia

While opiates are the most useful drugs for controlling severe pain, there are other therapies which may be indicated for special types of pain and which may be used in addition to, or as an adjunct to, opiates.

Bone pain

This usually arises from bone metastases from primary cancer of the lung, breast, prostate or thyroid, although other tumours may metastasize into bone; and of course primary malignancy may occur in bone as well. The pain is a dull, boring sensation, exacerbated by movement and pressure.

Radiotherapy is the most effective treatment as, apart from relieving pain, it can produce regression. Non-steroidal anti-inflammatory drugs act as anti-prostaglandins within the bone and are often very effective in relieving bone pain. Of the many drugs available the most useful are Froben [flurbiprofen] 50 mg − 100 mg tds (also available as 100 mg suppositories and sustained release capsules 200 mg), and Indocid [indomethacin] 25 mg − 50 mg tds (also available as 100 mg suppositories and as sustained release tablets 75 mg). Both these drugs may cause gastric irritation, in which case Benoral [benorylate] 10 mls bd is useful and does not cause dyspeptic symptoms.

Steroids relieve bone pain by diminishing the inflammatory and oedematous reaction in and around the metastases, so reducing the tumour size. It is better to give steroids in the form of dexamethasone as larger doses should be given initially, such as dexamethasone 8 mg daily given with ranitidine 150 mg bd to prevent dyspepsia. Once pain relief is achieved the dose may be reduced gradually.

Immobilization is occasionally helpful, although patients do not usually welcome plaster or splints.

Visceral pain

If it is a pain like colic, it is due to partial obstruction in the intestine, urinary tract or biliary tract. Large doses of opiates may be needed but the addition of anti-spasmodics is very helpful, such as Pro-Banthine [propantheline] 15 mg tds, Merbentyl [dicyclomine] 10 mg or 20 mg tds or Buscopan [hyoscine butyl-bromide] 10 mg − 20 mg tds (also available as injection 20 mg which can be added to diamorphine in the syringe driver). Continued use of these drugs may produce troublesome side effects such as dry mouth or urinary retention.

If the pain is continuous it may be due to an enlarged liver or other abdominal viscera. Large doses of steroids help this type of pain. Start with dexamethasone in a dose of at least 12 mg daily.

Muscle spasm

This can be extremely painful. The treatment can include: physiotherapy and sometimes splinting, Lioresal [baclofen] tablets 10 mg tds (gradually increasing as required, maximum 100 mg qds), Rivotril [clonazepam] 0.5 mg and 2 mg tablets (0.5 mg bd gradually increasing as required, maximum 8 mg daily), Dantrium [dantrolene] 25 mg and 100 mg tablets (25 mg tds gradually increasing as required, maximum 100 mg qds), Carisoma [carisoprodol] 125 mg and 350 mg tablets (125 mg tds increasing as required to 350 mg tds). Nocturnal cramps are occasionally helped by quinine sulphate 300 mg nocte. Peripheral spasm may be helped by nerve blocks.

Nerve compression

Strong analgesic medication is often inadequate to give complete relief from severe neuritic pains caused by nerve compression. Diuretics and steroids are useful co-analgesics but the only really effective treatment lies in a consideration of how the painful sensations are transmitted.

Transcutaneous electric nerve stimulation [TENS]

The gate theory of pain suggests that stimulation of large afferent nerve fibres reduces the input from peripheral pain receptors to the brain. It is also postulated that endogenous opiates produced by TENS assist analgesia. TENS is produced from a portable, battery powered stimulator giving high frequency, low voltage stimuli through the skin to the peripheral nerves. Optimum siting of the electrodes and adjustment of the stimulator may not be obtained at once, and there is scope for trial, with the help of the patient, to obtain the best result. While TENS occasionally produces dramatic improvement, the results are variable. As a non-invasive means of relieving pain TENS can be a useful alternative to analgesic medication. A complete TENS system costs between £60 and £90.

Nerve blocks

Ablation of a nerve pathway can be achieved by a neurolytic injection of diluted phenol or alcohol. This needs the help of an expert, usually an anaesthetist, as the injection needs to be pinpointed accurately. A trial injection of a local anaesthetic is used initially and if this is effective full ablation is then performed. A successful block will give permanent relief of pain allowing gradual reduction, and even complete withdrawal, of analgesic medication. The commonest blocks are sympathetic, epidural, intra-thecal, coeliac, brachial plexus. In suitable patients the results can be dramatic.

Some blocks may produce permanent, partial or even complete paresis of a limb, or sometimes urinary or bowel incontinence. Patients must be warned beforehand if there is a risk of these side effects, in case they consider that the possibility of permanent loss of mobility or control, is too high a price to pay for complete pain relief.

Tender 'trigger points' or intercostal pain may be relieved by local infiltration with a mixture of Depo-Medrone [methylprednisolone acetate] 1 ml mixed with 1% Xylocaine 2 ml.

Procedures such as neurosurgery (cordotomy or thalamotomy) or pituitary ablation may be considered for intractable pain, but these extreme measures are very rarely indicated.

Case history

Four years ago when Mr. P. retired, he and his wife went to live in a warmer country. They were enjoying their retirement until nine months ago, when Mrs. P. began to complain of low back and deep pelvic pains. The local doctor treated this as a musculo-skeletal condition and arranged for physiotherapy. However, exercises exacerbated the discomfort which gradually became more disabling. After six months, with no sign of improvement, they returned to London for further advice. X-rays revealed scattered metastases in the lumbo-sacral spine and right side of the pelvis, and biopsy confirmed that these were malignant deposits from an unidentified bowel primary. Radiotherapy gave some relief but after three months, during which she developed weakness of her right leg, she was admitted to St. Joseph's Hospice. On admission, she was in excruciating pain in the right pelvis, exacerbated even by slight movement. There was local bone tenderness and also severe neuritic pain radiating to the right ankle. She had been taking MST Continus 10 mg bd with no relief. She also had retention of urine, with bladder up to the umbilicus, and flaccid paresis of the right leg. She was treated with oral morphine which was rapidly increased in dosage over the first four days to 40 mg four hourly. She was also given non-steroidal anti-inflammatory treatment in the form of Froben (flurbiprophen) 100 mg tds, dexamethasone 12 mg daily, and a catheter was inserted. There was significant but inadequate pain relief from this treatment. Accordingly, an intra-thecal nerve block was performed. This procedure gave her complete relief from pain and she remained pain-free in the three months after it was performed. The doses of morphine and dexamethasone were reduced. She was up in a chair for most of the day, busy with various handicrafts and completely relaxed, although her general condition slowly weakened and she died peacefully with no recurrence of pain.

The technique for this patient's intra-thecal block was: lumbar puncture at levels of L1/L2 and L2/L3; free flow of C.S.F.; 0.8 ml of 5% phenol and glycerin injected at each level. The patient was supine with the left hip raised and this position was maintained for 4 hours.

Neuralgia

This unpleasant pain is common in malignancy, affecting the head and neck. While analgesics already described are needed, in addition the following are particularly useful: Tegretol [carbamazepine] 200 mg tablet (starting dose 200 mg bd increasing as required to 400 mg qds), amitriptyline 25 mg − 100 mg nocte and Epilim [sodium valproate] (starting dose 200 mg bd increasing as required to 400 mg tds).

Raised intracranial pressure

This causes severe headache, neck rigidity and vomiting as well as neurological defects.

If the symptoms are due to intracranial malignancy, a trial of steroids in high doses is well worthwhile. Steroids act by reducing the amount of fluid in and around tumours thereby reducing their size, and so diminishing intracranial pressure. Not all tumours are responsive. Dexamethasone may be used as a therapeutic trial in a dose of 16 mg or 20 mg daily. Any response will be evident within a few days, and if there is no response within six days, the dexamethasone should be discontinued. If it is used for a longer period withdrawal should be gradual.

If there is a response (and the response is occasionally dramatic), the dexamethasone should be continued, although the dose will have to be reduced gradually otherwise Cushingoid features will develop. The reduction of dosage will have to be empirical, and the level of dose will depend on balancing the benefit against any side effects from the dexamethasone.

When patients are on continual high doses of dexamethasone it is wise to give ranitidine 150 mg bd concurrently to prevent gastric irritation. Regular testing for glycosuria and hyperglycaemia is advisable. There is also a tendency to develop fungus infections especially in the mouth [oral thrush] (see p. 39).

As the tumour continues to increase in size, the symptoms of raised intracranial pressure will return despite the steroid. When this happens the symptoms should be treated by analgesics and anti-emetics. In general the non-steroidal anti-inflammatory drugs and benzodiazepines are more useful than opiates for the headaches and neck rigidity of raised intracranial pressure.

Infection and ulceration

Cellulitis and abscesses should be treated with appropriate antibiotics, and surgical drainage may be necessary. Sores, ulcers and fungating lesions can be extremely painful. To assist in treating these, short acting opiates such as Palfium [dextromoramide] one or two tablets fifteen minutes before a drainage procedure, should be given. If more severe discomfort is anticipated, intravenous diazepam 10 mg or inhalation of nitrous oxide and oxygen via Entonox apparatus is also helpful.

Other causes of pain

A dying patient may suffer great distress from conditions quite unrelated to the terminal disease such as toothache, musculo-skeletal conditions, thrombophlebitis, constipation, haemorrhoids and various infections. They should respond to specific treatment and such treatment should not be withheld just because the patient is dying.

Nausea and vomiting

There are many causes of nausea and vomiting, and the patient may feel ill and weak with dizziness, headaches and sweating. Causes include drugs (such as opiates, digoxin, cytotoxics, oestrogens, steroids, non-steroidal anti-inflammatories); radiotherapy; biochemical causes (such as hypercalcaemia and uraemia); infections (such as urinary tract infection); gastric irritation (such as a stomach tumour); hepatic metastases; intestinal obstruction; severe constipation; raised intracranial pressure; vestibular disturbance; coughing; and fear and anxiety.

Drugs suspected of causing nausea and vomiting should be withdrawn if possible. If they are essential, they should be given in a form to diminish their nauseating propensity, for example prednisolone can be given with an enteric coating.

Gastric irritation

This can be relieved by mist mag trisil co 10 ml tds, Asilone tablets or suspension, Gaviscon tablets to chew or liquid 10 ml bd, or Pyrogastrone tablets to chew.

Oesophageal reflux

Suitable preparations are Mucaine suspension 10 ml ac, Tagamet (cimetidine) 200 mg tds and 400 mg nocte, and Zantac (ranitidine) 15 mg bd or 300 mg nocte.

Hypercalcaemia

This should be suspected where there are bone metastases and the patient is vomiting and confused. Large doses of steroids by injection help, but they are unreliable. Phosphate-Sandoz 1 tds helps milder cases. The most effective treatment is with diphosphonates adopting the following procedure:

Controlling dehydration with IV saline 3 litres in 24 hours; subcutaneous injection of salmon calcitonin 100 iu bd for two days; Didronel (diphosphonate) 7.5 mg for each kg of body weight, given daily as an IV infusion, diluted with at least 250 ml of normal saline for three days, and oral Didronel 20 mg per kg of body weight, given daily on an empty stomach thereafter.

Vomiting from cerebral causes

Dexamethasone 4 mg qid as tablets or injection should be given for two weeks then the dose should gradually be reduced to 2 to 4 mg daily. Ranitidine 300 mg nocte should be used whenever dexamethasone is prescribed.

This treatment reduces tumour oedema but the improvement may only last for a few weeks (occasionally for several months in slow growing tumours) as the tumour itself continues to grow. Remission of symptoms resulting from the administration of dexamethasone is only temporary, and when the symptoms return there is little purpose in continuing the dexamethasone.

Intestinal obstruction

This is usually impossible to relieve by surgery in terminal illness, although it may be considered in appropriate cases, for example if it is thought that the patient may have several months to live and is willing to undergo surgery.

Pain and nausea are treated by analgesic and anti-emetic drugs which may be given per rectum or by injection. If injections are needed regularly the drugs may be given via a Graseby syringe driver. The patient may continue to vomit once or twice a day but the pain and constant nausea can be relieved by appropriate medication.

The peristalsis-stimulating anti-emetics, Maxolon and Motilium, should not be used for vomiting caused by intestinal obstruction. Buscopan (hyoscine

Choice of Anti-emetics

Groups/drugs	Dose	Formulations available	Notes
Antihistamines			
cyclizine (Valoid)	50 mg tds	tabs/inj	
promethazine (Phenergan)	25 mg tds	tabs/liquid/inj	All cause drowsiness
dimenhydrinate (Dramamine)	100 mg tds	tabs	
Butyrophenones			
droperidol (Droleptan)	10 mg tds	tabs/liquid/inj	Useful after chemotherapy
haloperidol (Serenace)	0.5 – 1.5 mg tds	tabs/liquid/inj	Wide variety of presentation including drops. Prolonged use may cause extra-pyramidal effects
Phenothiazines			
prochloperazine (Stemetil)	5 – 10 mg 4 hourly tds	tabs/inj/liquid supps	Large doses or long-term use can cause dyskinesia – patient appears fidgety. Improves when dose lowered
promazine (Sparine)	25 mg tds	liquid/inj	
chlorpromazine (Largactil)	10 – 25 mg tds or 100 mg supp	tabs/liquid/inj/ supps	Also cause dry mouth which is dose related
methotrimeprazine (Veractil/Nozinan)	25 mg tds	tabs/inj	
Anticholinergics			
hyoscine	0.4 mg	tabs/inj	Effective but causes dry mouth and blurring of vision
butylbromide (Buscopan)	10 – 20 mg tds	tabs/inj	Useful for gastro-intestinal spasm
Dopamine antagonists			
metoclopramide (Maxolon/Gastrobid Continus)	5 – 10 mg tds or 15 mg SR bd	tabs/liquid/inj and slow release tabs	Increases gastric emptying and gastro-oesophageal sphincter tone – also centrally acting
domperidone (Motilium)	10 mg tds	tabs/suspension/ supps	Similar to metoclopramide

If one drug is not effective a combination of drugs from different groups can be used. It may be necessary to administer anti-emetics via a syringe driver for persistent vomiting butylbromide) 20 mg by injection is useful for both pain and vomiting of intestinal obstruction. It may be included with other medication in the syringe driver in a daily dose of 40 mg.

Naso-gastric tubes and intravenous fluid are nearly always unnecessary but it is important to maintain mouth care and moisturization of mucous membranes.

Fear and anxiety

If emotional tension is thought to be a cause of nausea and vomiting appropriate anxiolytics are Valium (diazepam) 2 to 5 mg tds (this is also available in syrup and injections or suppositories 5 or 10 mg), or Ativan (lorazepam) 1 mg bd (this is also available as a 2.5 tablet or 4 mg injection).

If depression is suspected use Bolvidon (mianserin) 30 to 60 mg nocte or amitriptyline 50 to 75 mg nocte.

Anorexia

This is a common complaint of patients with advanced cancer. Its causes include drugs e.g. cytotoxics, nausea and vomiting and fear of vomiting, gastrointestinal abnormalities or constipation, jaundice, biochemical changes such as uraemia or hypercalcaemia, anxiety and depression and sore or dry mouth.

The various tonics which can be prescribed have little effect. The most useful drugs are corticosteroids. Prednisolone (preferably enteric-coated) 10 mg bd often produces a significant increase in appetite and a feeling of increased strength and well-being. Efficient mouth care is essential to eradicate soreness, especially due to thrush and dryness. Small doses of antidepressant drugs, e.g. Bolvidon (mianserin) 20 mg nocte may elevate the patient's mood and increase appetite, but antidepressants do not produce significant improvement in less than ten days. Small doses of anxiolytic drugs, e.g. Valium (diazepam) or Ativan (lorazepam) will help anxiety.

Meals should be attractively presented in small quantities and prepared in accordance with the patient's taste. An alcoholic aperitif is often helpful.

Sore and dry mouth

This can be caused by fungus infections (thrush), dental problems such as ill-fitting dentures, decaying teeth or dental abscess, aphthous ulceration, drugs (such as cytotoxics, phenothiazines, tricyclic antidepressants), vitamin deficiency, herpes, blood dyscrasias, diabetes, local radiotherapy, mouth breathing, dehydration and cancrum oris.

Routine mouth care is an essential nursing procedure in terminal illness, and should include the administration of mouthwashes using glycerin and thymol, Oraldene, hydrogen peroxide or Difflam Oral Rinse.

Fungal infection

This is common and if not eradicated it may become systemic. It should be treated by using Nystan oral suspension 2 ml four hourly (dentures should be rinsed with Nystan also), Nystan Pastilles, Fungilin (amphotericin) lozenges, Pimafucin suspension 1% 10 drops after meals, Daktarin gel (miconazole 25 mg/ml) 10 ml held in mouth as long as possible qid, Nizoral (ketoconazole) 200 mg bd in tablets or suspension or Diflucan (fluconazole) 50 mg capsule daily.

Dental problems

The patient's cachexia may cause shrinkage of the gums, and dentures then become loose and irritating. Other dental problems may also need the attention of a dentist and even though life expectancy may be only a matter of a few weeks, dental care may provide much appreciated comfort for the patient.

Aphthous ulceration

Local applications of Medilave Gel (cetylpyridinium), Adcortyl or Orabase (triamcinolone oral paste), Bioral (carbenoxolone sodium) or AAA (local anaesthetic) Spray.

Drugs

Those drugs suspected of causing mouth soreness should be withdrawn or the dosage reduced. Cytotoxic drugs frequently cause gingivitis or glossitis. Antibiotics occasionally do likewise. Tricyclic antidepressants, phenothiazines, antihistamines and anticholinergics all cause dryness of the mouth, but this is usually dose related.

Vitamin deficiency

Soreness of the mouth does occasionally respond to vitamin therapy especially vitamin B complex and vitamin C, and these are worth trying.

Herpes

Herpid (idoxuridine 5%) applied for four days at the first sign of infection, Symmetrel (amantadine) 100 mg bd or Zovirax (acyclovir) 200 mg 5 times a day can be used for treatment. Quadruple the dose of Zovirax for herpes zoster.

Blood dyscrasias

It is not usually appropriate or possible to give specific treatment for these in terminal cancer, although occasionally after considering all the relevant factors concerning a particular patient, a blood transfusion may be given.

Diabetes

This may develop in pancreatic disease or as a result of high doses of steroids. If it is due to the latter, reducing the dose of steroids is usually effective. Insulin or oral hypoglycaemics may occasionally be necessary.

Mouth dryness

This can be caused by local radiotherapy, dehydration or breathing through the mouth and should be treated by giving the patient chopped ice, flavoured according to their taste, frequent ice cold drinks, sweets to suck, pineapple to chew or a moisturizing drink which provides artificial saliva. This can be made from methylcellulose 2.5 g with an acceptable flavouring such as tincture of orange or lemon essence and diluted with 300 ml of water. Frequent small sips of this drink reduce the sensation of dryness. Foam stick applicators are useful for applying fluid and medication to the mouth and tongue.

Cancrum oris

The mouth may become grossly ulcerated producing a foul discharge and constant soreness. The patient is reluctant to accept any food, drink or medication by mouth. This condition needs intensive nursing care with half hourly oral toilet using hydrogen peroxide. The methylcellulose drink described above can be given, vitamin B complex, vitamin C, Flagyl (metronidazole) 400 mg tds and Nystan 2 ml four hourly.

Dysphagia

This condition is caused by sore and dry mouth, pharyngeal obstruction, oesophageal obstruction (due to tumour, ulceration or stricture), neuromuscular disease (as may occur in motor neurone disease), central neurological failure (as in bulbar palsy) and fungal infection.

Treatment is by dexamethasone 4 mg qid by injection. Other medication should be given via a syringe driver or by rectal suppositories, and intensive mouth care and moisturizing of the mouth is essential. If the dysphagia has been caused by a fungal infection spreading down the oesophagus, anti-fungal treatment such as Nystan oral suspension should be given.

Even in advanced cases the insertion of a Celestin Tube may be possible if the obstruction is in the lower third of the oesophagus. An IV infusion may be needed to relieve distressing dehydration in patients with neuromuscular dysphagia or for total organic dysphagia when the patient's condition is not terminal.

Constipation

This is a frequent concomitant of terminal illness. Impacted faeces may simulate abdominal malignancy. Once this impaction is relieved and bowel mobility restored, the patient's condition frequently improves dramatically.

Causes are inactivity, weakness and diminished intake of food. Constipation may also result as a side effect of medication, such as opiates or anticholinergics.

Treatment is by Dulcolax (bisacodyl) suppositories 10 mg, manual removal of impacted faeces lubricated with a local anaesthetic such as Xylocaine Gel. This may require light anaesthesia by intravenous Valium or inhalation of nitrous oxide and oxygen from an Entonox machine. High impaction may be relieved by an arachis oil enema to be retained for as long as possible.

Laxatives

Once impaction has been eliminated normal bowel activity should be encouraged by using bowel stimulants, bulk stimulants, lubricants, faecal softeners or osmotic laxatives either separately or in various combinations.

Bowel stimulants:

sennoside (senna) 7.5 mg tablets − 2 to 4 tablets at night, also available as granules and syrup

Laxoberal (sodium picosulphate) 5 to 15 ml nocte

Dulcolax (bisacodyl) 5 mg tablets or 5 mg or 10 mg suppositories

Prostigmin (neostigmine) 15 mg tablet is also useful but should not be used if organic intestinal obstruction is suspected

Bulk stimulants:
    bran
    Cologel (methylcellulose) 459 mg/5 ml with fluid
    Celevac (methylcellulose) 500 mg tablet with sodium bicarbonate
    Fybogel 3.5 granules in sachet with fluid
    Normacol granules 2 × 5 ml spoonfuls bd with fluid
    Regulan (ispaghula husk 3.6 g) one sachet tds
Lubricants:
    liquid paraffin (often mixed with other laxatives such as Agarol or Milpar)
    glycerine suppositories
Faecal softeners:
    Dioctyl (dioctyl sodium sulphosuccinate) 100 mg tablet and syrup
    Normax (co-danthrusate)
Osmotic laxatives:
    Duphalac (lactulose) 15 ml bd
    Fletchers' phosphate enema
The larger dose of these various laxatives is needed in terminal illness. The bulk stimulants are less frequently used as patients are often reluctant to take copious fluid. It does help, however, if the patient can be persuaded to take extra fluid, particularly fruit drinks.

Diarrhoea

This is less common than constipation in advanced cancer.

Causes are drugs such as some antibiotics, pancreatic tumours, the effects of radiotherapy, tumours of the large intestine, or anxiety and nervous tension. A frequent condition is spurious diarrhoea which is due to the ball-valve effect of rock hard faeces and is essentially constipation. It resolves when the hard lumps are evacuated as a result of enemas and purgatives.

Treatment is by codeine phosphate 15 mg tds; Lomotil (diphenoxylate HCl 2.5 mg and atropine sulphate 0.025) 2 to 4 tablets qid. Codeine phosphate and Lomotil have an opiate-like action and are usually very effective.

Imodium (loperamide HCL 2 mg) 2 tds also available as a syrup, inhibits peristalsis.

Steroid retention enemas (Predsol or Predenema) are very useful for persistent diarrhoea caused by radiotherapy or tumour infiltration.

Colifoam (hydrocortisone acetate 10%) rectal insertion bd using an applicator.

Bulky offensive stools of steatorrhoea associated with pancreatic tumours: Pancrex V (pancreatin/protease/lipase and amylase) available as capsules or tablets given with food.

Diarrhoea is occasionally due to fear or anxiety and can be relieved by mild tranquillizers, e.g. Valium (diazepam) 2 mg tds or Ativan (lorazepam) 1 mg bd.

Micturition problems

Retention

This can be caused by drugs such as the anticholinergics (e.g. propantheline), the sympathomimetics (e.g. ephedrine) and the tricyclic antidepressants; neurological problems such as paraplegia; an organic obstruction such as an enlarged prostate; tumour infiltration or constipation.

To treat urinary retention it is usually necessary to pass a catheter, although if impacted constipation is the problem, relieving this may render catheterization unnecessary.

Incontinence

This is a humiliating symptom, producing acute distress. It is caused by drugs such as diuretics; infection; neurological problems; urinary fistulae or anxiety.

Specific treatment should be given as appropriate but catheterization is usually necessary. Valium (diazepam) and Ativan (lorazepam) are useful in cases of anxiety.

Infections

These are frequent. The first sign of a urinary tract infection may be apparently unrelated to the urinary tract, i.e. confusion, rigor, headache, hyperpyrexia, sweating, vomiting. They usually respond to an appropriate antibiotic and a broad spectrum antibiotic may be given whilst awaiting the result of sensitivity investigations in the laboratory, such as Ipral (trimethoprim) 200 mg bd; Amoxil (amoxycillin) 500 mg tds; Mictral (nalidixic acid) 660 mg sachet tds; Distaclor (cefaclor) 250 mg tds and Ciproxin (ciprofloxaxin) 500 mg to 750 mg bd.

Painful urethral spasm is helped by Urispas (flavoxate) 100 mg 2 tds or Pro-Banthine (propantheline) 15 mg tds.

Catheterization

There should be no hesitation in passing a catheter for a patient in terminal illness who is suffering from frequency, incontinence or recurrent retention. A uridom is a useful alternative for male patients with incontinence. As long as the purpose and procedure is explained beforehand patients are usually willing to accept catheterization. A self-retaining silastic catheter may be left *in situ* for several months.

Bladder wash-outs

These are not a routine necessity, but are helpful should there be problems with drainage caused, for example, by debris. Hibitane (chlorhexidine) 1/5000 can be used and the Uro-Tainer series of bladder irrigations are very useful. Bladder haemorrhage may be reduced by daily bladder washes using 0.01% silver nitrate solution. Dicynene may also help.

Haemorrhage

The instinctive reaction of doctors and nurses is to do everything possible to stop the bleeding, but this is not always the appropriate treatment in terminal illness, nor are resuscitation or transfusions generally used. However, patients and relatives are alarmed by any bleeding, and even small amounts of blood seeping through dressings stain clothes and bedding very quickly.

Small haemorrhages from problems such as fungating lesions, may be effectively controlled by cautery or astringent application such as silver nitrate 0.5% lotion or pads of gauze soaked in adrenaline 1/1000 or acetone. Radiotherapy may also help. Dicynene (ethamsylate) 500 mg qid is often very helpful in reducing small vessel haemorrhage.

A massive haemorrhage may be heralded by small prodromal bleeds. This also applies to haemorrhage from internal organs. Haemoptysis, haematemesis or malaena may be slight at first but may be a warning of a massive haemorrhage to come. Radiotherapy may diminish a haemoptysis and steroid retention enemas may diminish bleeding from the rectum and colon. If a large haemorrhage is anticipated, bright red towels and drapes should be available, and a suction machine ready for immediate use should be adjacent to the patient. Opiates, preferably diamorphine by injection, in an adequate dose (taking account of the dosage of opiates the patient is already receiving) should be given immediately a massive haemorrhage occurs.

Pressure sores

These develop through four stages — hyperaemia, blistering, broken skin and penetration. Blistering and broken skin are painful, while hyperaemia and penetration are not usually painful unless there is some infection.

Pressure sores can be prevented. The skin should be oiled regularly using Oilatum (arachis oil 21%), Balneum Oilatum Emollient (wood alcohol and liquid paraffin) 15 ml in a bath, Vaseline, Conotrane Cream or Sprilon Barrier Spray. The patient should be encouraged to move frequently to relieve pressure on areas of skin likely to become sore such as heels, elbows, toes, sacrum etc. Protection of these areas can also be given by sheepskins to lie on and sheepskin heel pads. There are also several special beds available such as the Ripple, Simpson and Net beds which relieve pressure.

If pressure sores do become established the first procedure is to deslough and excise dead tissue. The sore should be cleansed and packed if needed with eusol and glycerin, eusol and liquid paraffin, hydrogen peroxide 3% or Betadine cream or paint. The Silastic Foam Dressing is very useful for deep excavated sores. Light anaesthesia such as from nitrous oxide and oxygen via Entonox, or Stesolid (diazepam) 10 mg per rectum may be needed when applying dressings.

When infections and/or cellulitis are present take a swab for sensitivity and give the appropriate antibiotic systemically. Antibiotics or steroid creams applied locally are not effective. If the sore is very painful Xylocaine Gel may be applied around the edges. Infra-red treatment will improve circulation and aid healing. The deeper sores may harbour anaerobic organisms and should be treated with hydrogen peroxide packs and with Flagyl (metronidazole) 400 mg tds given orally. Skin grafting and surgical procedures are usually not relevant in terminal illness.

Skin irritation

The threshold for this varies with the patient's mood and morale. When it is severe it causes great distress and misery. Causes include drug and food sensitivity, external irritants such as appliances or antiseptics, fungus infections, jaundice, eczema, scabies, extreme dryness of the skin and herpes.

For treatment apply Oilatum cream (arachis oil 21%) to the dry skin or add Balneum Oilatum Emollient 15 ml to the bath. This treatment moisturizes the skin. Alpha Keri (mineral oil and lanolin oil) can be used in the same way.

Pruritis soon subsides when internal or external sensitizing agents are withdrawn, and steroid creams are usually very soothing.

Fungus infections, especially in the inguinal and perineal regions are common and the skin around a colostomy may also be affected by fungal infections. These can be treated by 1% Canesten (clotrimazole cream) or 1% Ecostatin (econazole cream). Diflucan (fluconazole) 50 mg capsule daily or Nizoral (ketoconazole) 200 mg bd may be necessary to clear gut infection.

The pruritis of jaundice may be helped by steroids such as prednisolone 10 mg bd, Questran (cholestyramine) 4 mg qid, antihistamines such as Piriton (chlorpheniramine) 4 mg tds or Phenergan (promethazine) 25 mg tds. Rifampcin 600 mg daily is also helpful.

The appearance and distribution of the rash might suggest the possibility of scabies which soon responds to specific treatment.

Herpetic lesions respond to local applications of Herpid (idoxuridine 5%) during the vesicular stage. Zovirax (acyclovir) tablets 200 mg 5 times a day and Zovirax cream are effective treatments, but for herpes zoster use Zovirax tablets 800 mg 5 times daily.

Hyperhidrosis or excessive sweating is often present in advanced cancer. It may respond to Indocid (indomethacin) 25 mg tds or as a suppository 100 mg nocte or Inderal (propranolol) 40 mg tds.

Fungating lesions

If lesions are infected, systemic antibiotics will help once sensitivity has been established. Local antibiotics are not effective. Flagyl (metronidazole) 400 mg tds is useful to control the foul smelling discharge due to anaerobic infection. The lesion should first be cleansed with eusol and liquid paraffin or Hibitane (chlorhexidine) 1/1000 or Betadine (povidone iodine) as a paint, spray or ointment. Persistent bleeding points may be cauterized or covered with pads soaked in adrenaline 1/1000 or acetone. Dicynene may sometimes help.

Some breast fungations will regress considerably with hormone therapy such as Nolvadex (tamoxifen) 20 mg daily or Farlutal (medroxyprogesterone) 250 mg qid. Radiotherapy is effective for larger lesions which have not already been irradiated. Exceptionally surgery may be considered.

Smell

A foul disagreeable smell emanating from the patient is a personal embarrassment, unpleasant for relatives and visitors, for other patients and also for those caring for the patient. The usual causes are fungating lesions, infected discharges from pressure sores or fistulae, steatorrhoea or cancrum oris and nasopharyngeal infections.

External lesions should be cleansed with eusol, hydrogen peroxide, Betadine (povidone iodine) or Hibitane (chlorhexidine). Swabs should be taken from infected discharges and an appropriate antibiotic should be given systematically after sensitivity tests. Anaerobic organisms produce foul smelling discharges and are prevalent in deep sores and fistulae. Hydrogen peroxide lavage is helpful and Flagyl (metronidazole) tablets 400 mg tds should be given orally.

Steatorrhoea causes bulky offensive faeces and arises from deficient pancreatic secretions. It may be helped by giving Pancrex V (pancreatin, protease, lipase and amylase) 2 capsules with food qid.

Cancrum oris requires intensive oral hygiene using Oraldene, glycerin and thymol or hydrogen peroxide mouthwashes, antifungal lozenges (Fungilin) and

Nystan suspension. Flagyl (metronidazole) tablets 400 mg tds also help and vitamin B complex is often effective.

Air fresheners may be used discreetly and deodorants such as Nilodor, de Roma and Dor should be applied to dressings.

Weakness and tiredness

The cachexia of terminal illness produces a lethargy and feebleness which is very frustrating. Even minor activities require a major effort. Tonics are not effective but corticosteroids such as enteric-coated prednisolone 10 mg bd are often helpful. Very rarely it may be appropriate to give a particular patient a blood transfusion if anaemia is the cause of the weakness. Small doses of CNS stimulants such as amphetamine which are now regarded as unsuitable for general use, may occasionally give considerable benefit to patients in terminal illness. For example, Dexedrine (dexamphetamine) 5 mg mane. Patients can also be provided with undemanding diversions such as simple craft work or 'talking books'.

Immobility and paresis

The frustrations of diminished autonomy produce a sense of helplessness and anger in having to be dependent on others for even minor personal requirements. This is particularly hard on those who have a proud or independent personality. Everything the patient needs or is expected to need should be placed within easy reach. Patients do not like to have to summon assistance for every minor requirement. There are a multitude of gadgets now available to assist handicapped and disabled patients and these should be provided and their use explained. The Disabled Living Foundation has a catalogue of useful aids, and advice can be obtained on equipment for the disabled (see Appendix 2).

Appropriate physiotherapy diminishes stiffness, maintains circulation and helps to prevent trophic lesions. Frequent turning and special chairs and beds are essential nursing procedures.

These patients need diversion and recreational activities compatible with their interests and capabilities.

Oedema

Localized oedema

This may be caused by tumour infiltrations interfering with venous return or lymphatic drainage. Unless there is generalized oedema as well, diuretics are not helpful and may even cause uncomfortable dehydration.

Generalized oedema

This is caused by anaemia, malnutrition, protein deficiency, renal failure, hepatic failure, myocardial failure or drugs such as steroids, for example Silboestrol.

Diuretics are often very helpful and frusemide is the most effective, and is an essential treatment for pulmonary oedema, preferably by IV injection. Moduretic (amiloride 5 mg with hydrochlorothiazide 60 mg) is also a useful diuretic. Digoxin should be prescribed with care as overdosage may cause unpleasant side effects.

Lymphoedema

A limb may become massively enlarged causing distressing heaviness and distension. At the first sign of oedema, rings should be removed from all fingers. A Jobst or Flowtron compression sleeve applied for about an hour each day will not cure the lymphoedema but will usually prevent the condition from developing to uncomfortable and unmanageable proportions. The limb should be supported in an elevated position and firm bandaging is also helpful. Steroids such as dexamethasone 4 mg bd are occasionally effective for local oedema. Anticoagulant treatment may be required for deep vein thrombosis.

Ascites

This only needs treatment if it is causing discomfort such as distension or dyspnoea. The patient is catheterized and the abdomen is then tapped allowing the ascitic fluid to drain slowly. Sudden decompression should be avoided. Injection of Coparavax (*Corynebacterium parvum*) 7 mg ampoule diluted and injected into the peritoneal cavity after draining the ascites is effective in preventing recurrence in about 60% of cases.

Dyspnoea

Causes are asthma, pulmonary oedema, infection, painful chest lesions, tumour infiltration, pleural effusion, pneumothorax, ascites, respiratory paresis, biochemical, anaemia and anxiety.

Treatment is by oxygen if the onset is sudden or until other medication has had time to work. It is not recommended or necessary for prolonged use.

Drugs: bronchodilators such as Ventolin (salbutamol) in tablets, syrup, inhaler or injection; aminophylline in suppositories or injection; diuretics such as Lasix (frusemide) in tablets or injection; steroids, i.e. prednisolone, dexamethasone in tablets, hydrocortisone, dexamethasone by injection; Becotide (beclomethasone) by inhalation.

Antibiotics should be used if this treatment is thought to be appropriate. They are often useful symptomatically if phlegm is thick or purulent. Chloramphenicol is a useful broad spectrum antibiotic since resistance is uncommon and the rare blood dyscrasias can be disregarded.

Opiates reduce the sensitivity of the respiratory centre to hypoxia and so reduce the subjective unpleasantness of the dyspnoea, but they must be given regularly. They also reduce pain associated with respiration from problems such as pleural rub or fractured ribs.

Atropine or hyoscine 0.4 to 0.6 mg by injection reduce secretions and are particularly useful in the final few hours.

Tranquillizers such as Valium (diazepam) 2 mg tds and Ativan (lorazepam) 1 mg tds reduce anxiety and improve muscle relaxation.

Steam inhalations, with or without the addition of Friar's Balsam (benzoin) or Karval capsules, are useful when phlegm is thick or for tracheo-laryngitis. Inhalation of a local anaesthetic such as 0.5% Marcain via a Bird Nebulizer or Pulmosonic inhaler anaesthetizes the lung receptors which are situated in the alveoli and also other receptors in the bronchioles and trachea. The result is a reduction of the subjective sensation of breathlessness. This is also very useful for the chronic unproductive cough which occurs in tracheo-laryngitis. Alevaire (tyloxapol 0.125%) may be given as an inhalation through a pressurized nebulizer to soften tenaceous sputum.

Other treatments are radiotherapy which reduces tumour size but care must be taken as, initially, it may increase oedema around the tumour. Blood transfusion is only of use on rare occasions. It may be considered if the patient's condition proves to be less advanced than it was thought to be at first. Patients in the terminal phase do not usually respond to transfusions and most do not like them. Aspiration of a pleural effusion is occasionally helpful for dyspnoea. In general patients do not like this and the procedure should only be undertaken after explaining it to the patient.

If ascites is large, tense and impeding diaphragmatic mobility the withdrawal of ascitic fluid may give dramatic relief to a dyspnoeic patient. Physiotherapy and breathing exercises are also very useful.

The dyspnoea threshold can be raised by giving the patient ample opportunities to express fears and anxieties. Give sympathy, understanding, diversion and encourage relaxation. The most distressing type of dyspnoea is that associated with anxiety and fear. These patients are dramatically improved by an appropriate anxiolytic such as Valium (diazepam) 10 mg orally or as suppository or by injection or Ativan (lorazepam) 1 mg or 2 mg orally or by injection.

Obstruction of the superior vena cava due to mediastinal tumour causes unpleasant cyanosis and oedema of the head, neck and upper limbs and severe dyspnoea. The best treatment is palliative radiotherapy which should be arranged urgently, dexamethasone 8 mg tds gradually reduced to 8 mg daily is also effective.

Cough

This can be caused by external irritants such as fumes, dust, smoke; inflammation (tracheitis, laryngitis, tumour infiltration); bronchospasm; seepage of fluid from lesions in the nose, mouth or pharynx; infections (bronchitis) and pulmonary oedema.

Many patients request a cough linctus treatment but this is not particularly effective. If one is prescribed, codeine linctus is a suitable cough suppressant. Sips of hot drinks such as orange or blackcurrant juice are very soothing. Steam inhalations with or without the addition of Friar's Balsam (benzoin) or a Karvol inhalation capsule can be effective. Bronchodilators such as Ventolin (salbutamol) 4 mg tablets tds, as syrup or via a pressurized inhaler or Pulmosonic, and aminophylline as a slow release tablet (Phyllocontin Continus) 226 mg, or in the form of a suppository are also useful. A very effective treatment is the inhalation of a local anaesthetic such as Marcain delivered as an aerosol under positive pressure (see p. 50).

Opiates which may be given concomitantly for pain also help to diminish cough. If they are not already being given, small doses may be prescribed specifically for cough, e.g. Physeptone linctus (methadone 2 mg/5 ml).

Ephedrine and medications containing it should be avoided due to the risk of urinary retention.

A productive cough with mucopurulent sputum may be relieved by prescribing a broad spectrum antibiotic for a few days such as chloramphenicol 250 qid or Amoxil (amoxycillin) 500 mg tds.

The frothy expectoration of pulmonary oedema is helped by diuretics such as Lasix (frusemide) 40 mg bd or, if acute, by injection. A suction machine may be needed.

Physiotherapy, such as breathing exercises, chest percussion or postural drainage may be helpful. Most patients with a persistent cough feel more comfortable when propped up. If there are upper respiratory lesions causing a rhinorrhoea, measures may be needed to reduce the drip such as a steroid nasal spray (Beconase) or Rynacrom drops or spray.

Hiccough

This can be a very persistent and annoying complaint. It can be caused by diaphragmatic irritation as from tumour infiltration resulting in gastric or abdominal distension; phrenic nerve irritation; CNS tumour and metabolic disorders such as uraemia.

For treatment keep the patient propped up, give frequent small drinks and give peppermint sweets to suck. Largactil (chlorpromazine) 25 mg tds (larger doses if needed); Temazepam 10 mg nocte; Maxolon (metoclopramide) 10 mg qid hastens gastric emptying; Asilone suspension 10 ml bd and phenytoin 100 mg if a cerebral cause is suspected. A naso-gastric tube occasionally helps. Steroids are often very helpful but large doses are needed such as dexamethasone 4 mg tds until relief is obtained, then reduce slowly.

Nervous and emotional problems

Fear and anxiety in a patient are usually easy to recognize. The facies generally express their emotions. Some patients attempt to disguise their feelings by a fixed smile which does not illuminate their eyes, and there is often a tightening of the facial muscles, particularly of the forehead.

In depth discussion is often needed to identify the cause or causes of the tension, and these may prove to be quite different from what one might expect. There are so many factors interwoven which may include familial, financial or spiritual factors, guilt, anger, fear of dying or unrelieved physical symptoms. If these can be identified and discussed much of the fear may be dispersed. A useful device is to encourage the patient to live each day for what pleasures, joys and comforts can be achieved in that day. If possible the patient could keep a diary and record the enjoyments experienced day by day, looking always for the positive uplifting events. The chaplain or pastor and social worker have important roles in supporting the anxious and frightened patient.

Medication

From the large range of drugs available, those most used at St. Joseph's Hospice are Valium (diazepam) 2 mg to 5 mg bd or tds and Ativan (lorazepam) 1 mg bd.

Depression is less common than might be expected in terminal illness but its incidence increases in proportion to how long the terminal stage is protracted. It is not always easy to differentiate sadness from depression.

Anti-depressant drugs do not usually have any significant effect until the patient has been taking them for about a week. If there is any suspicion that the patient is becoming depressed an early start should be made with anti-depressants. In general, patients in terminal illness respond to the smaller doses. Tricyclic anti-depressants such an amitriptyline 25 mg to 75 mg nocte may be used but their tendency to cause drowsiness and a dry mouth is sometimes unacceptable. Bolvidon (mianserin) 20 mg or 30 mg nocte is a very useful drug with fewer side effects. Some patients may require larger doses. Monoamine oxide inhibitors (MAOIs) are best avoided.

Case history

Mr. J., aged 55, had been very successful at buying and selling property. Carcinoma of the larynx had been treated with surgery, radiotherapy and chemotherapy. On admission he had a naso-gastric tube and a tracheostomy. He had much discomfort with infection and thrush and considerable cervical pain, all of which were relieved by appropriate medication. Fully aware of his diagnosis and prognosis, he was miserable and withdrawn. There was no family support, he was a widower with no children.

He showed no interest in recreational activities until he saw another patient making rugs. She soon taught him what to do. We then saw why he had been successful in business. Although he could not talk, he arranged to be transferred to another room, he purchased his materials more cheaply than we could, he found people to assist him and to get orders, and in no time he had a thriving rug factory in his room. He was so busy he often waved away the drug trolley.

He wrote a letter to us saying he had never been happier in his life − a remarkable statement from a successful businessman, making rugs in a hospice and needing tubes to help him breathe and feed. He continued happily and contentedly for nine months, when he died peacefully in his sleep.

Not everyone would wish to spend the last few months of their lives making rugs, but it is important to study patients' interests, capabilities and wishes and do everything possible to provide whatever is appropriate.

Those who have, or have had religious convictions gain peace and tranquillity by having spiritual comfort and support from their pastors. Close co-operation between doctors, nurses and clergy can be very rewarding.

Case history

Mr. F., 65, in advanced stage of carcinoma of lung. Weak, but symptoms well controlled, and he was up and mobile, but morose and withdrawn and fully aware of the diagnosis and prognosis. One day I said to him, 'Is there anything at all you would like us to do to help you to be more relaxed?' His reply was that he would dearly like to see his family before he died. He was a Frenchman who had come over with General de Gaulle and after the war, married an English girl and settled in London where he had a good job. He made desultory attempts to contact his family but they had all left the family farm in the south of France and as his interests were all in the U.K., he did not persevere.

His daughter had died about five years previously. His wife had died a year ago and shortly afterwards he had developed his cancer. He now had no family in the U.K. − just a few friends − and he felt lonely.

He gave us the address of his old family home and we got in touch with the Hotel de Ville, the gendarmerie and the curé in the nearest town. Nobody knew of his family but they promised to make enquiries. A few days later, the gendarmerie telephoned and gave us a contact number. We followed this up, found a brother and told him about Mr. F. We arranged for two brothers to come and see Mr. F. and for the Marie Curie Foundation to pay their expenses.

The following Saturday morning I witnessed their arrival. They were almost a caricature of Frenchmen − berets, moustaches, clutching bottles of wine, roars of laughter and great Gallic excitement. Mr. F. was transported with joy. They stayed for three days and departed, sad, but still laughing. Mr. F. died three weeks later, relaxed and peaceful with a huge grin on his face.

Restoration of family contacts and reconciling family relationships are often time consuming and emotionally demanding, but are supremely worthwhile.

Confusion

A distressing symptom for patients, families and carers. There are three main causes, although confusion in the dying patient may be a mixture of all three.

Fear

This is exacerbated by isolation or a change of environment. It can be caused by a misperception of sights and sounds, especially at night and is worse in those with physical disability such as deafness, blindness or immobility. It should be pre-empted by company, explanation and support.

Delirium (acute brain syndrome)

This is potentially reversible as it is mostly due to a toxic irritation of neurones. It can range from mild confusion to gross psychosis with hallucinations, paranoia and negativism. Its onset may be rapid but if the cause can be identified and treated rigorously there may be complete recovery. Its causes include toxic, e.g. chest and urinary tract infections (frequently delirium is the first sign of a developing infection); biochemical, e.g. hypercalcaemia, diabetes, uraemia, dehydration, hypoxia; drugs, e.g. sensitivity, excessive doses, interactions or sudden withdrawal. Preferably a person familiar to the patient should be in charge of the situation and avoid crowding (a well briefed relative may be helpful). Gentle coaxing in a calm unruffled manner often obtains co-operation.

Staff should not argue and be offended by the patient's behaviour. Search for a cause and treat it effectively with broad spectrum antibiotics for an infection, IV fluid and Didronel for hypercalcaemia. All medication should be reviewed and enquiries about drugs taken previously (remember alcohol) should be made. Patients who have diabetes usually require much lower doses of insulin or hypoglycaemic drugs in terminal illness, and if these drugs are continued, hypoglycaemia with acute delirium may develop rapidly.

Dementia (organic brain syndrome)

This is not reversible as it is due to the destruction of neurones. Onset is insidious with progressive memory loss and personality change. Twenty per cent of those over 80 are affected to some degree. Patients are usually placid, sluggish and withdrawn, though they may be aggressive at times if something they want, or wish to do, is denied them. Progressive intellectual impairment leads to difficulty in communication, forgetting natural functions with consequent incontinence. Neurological deficiency follows with unco-ordination and inability to feed themselves. Eventually they become chairbound.

The main objective of treatment is to make the most of those neurones which have not been destroyed. Mental and physical stimulation should be provided and isolation avoided. Patients should be persuaded to do as much as possible for themselves. Mobility should be encouraged and physiotherapy offered if necessary. A good personal appearance should be maintained and regular checks on general health, especially sight and hearing be made. Self-neglect may allow insidious development of disease. The patients should be entertained individually or in groups with music and simple games; with encouragement of reminiscences with family photographs and talks about their earlier lives. If a patient is hypothyroid or Parkinsonian, specific treatment will help.

Dementia does not respond to drug treatment at all, indeed as there is a deficiency of active neurones, normal doses of psychotropic drugs may easily lead to over-sedation. Mild sedation may be required at night.

Drugs for the anxious confused patient are: Valium (diazepam) 5 mg or 10 mg orally or as suppositories, Ativan (lorazepam) 1 mg or 2 mg orally or by injection, and Heminevrin (chlormethiazole) syrup 5 ml or capsule 192 mg may be taken bd or tds and double dose nocte.

Other drugs used for the confused patient are: Largactil (chlorpromazine) 25 mg, 50 mg, 100 mg tds orally, as a suppository or by injection; Melleril (thioridazine) 25 mg, 50 mg or 100 mg tds orally or by injection; Serenace (haloperidol) 0.5 mg, 1.5 mg or 10 mg tds orally or by injection; and Sparine (promazine) 25 mg, 50 mg or 100 mg tds orally or by injection.

Mild confusion requires only the smaller doses. Severe confusion and agitation will need the maximum doses. Once the patient is stabilized the dose is then gradually reduced. Intramuscular injection of 5 ml Paraldehyde is occasionally indicated for a more severely disturbed patient.

Occasionally a patient may respond to the converse of the above treatment i.e. CNS stimulants such as Dexedrine (dexamphetamine) 5 mg mane.

Insomnia

Rather than prescribing hypnotics routinely it is wise to enquire why the patient is not able to sleep. Insomnia can be caused by a number of factors: pain, coughing, vomiting, itching, incontinence or fear of incontinence, depression, fear, and an uncomfortable environment (too hot, cold, noisy etc).

Having investigated all possible causes of insomnia and given specific treatment and reassurance as appropriate, there remain those patients who do need sedation. If a patient is already accustomed to a hypnotic and it works, there is no point in changing it.

Useful drugs for night sedation are: Normison, Temazepam 10 mg and 20 mg and Welldorm 650 mg (dichloralphenazone) available in a capsule or elixir.

If there is some confusion or agitation add: Heminevrin (chlormethiazole) syrup 10 ml nocte or Largactil (chlorpromazine) 25 mg or 50 mg tablet (also available as a syrup or 100 mg suppositories).

Disfigurement

This may cause enormous mental suffering. The feeling of being repulsive is demoralizing and causes the patient to reject human contact and seek isolation. Disfigurement is particularly distressing to women and young people. It may range from a single scar about which the patient is inordinately sensitive to a gross fungating lesion. Cosmetics, scar covering creams and sunglasses may conceal minor blemishes. A wig may work wonders for a patient with an unsightly scalp, for example after chemotherapy.

It is futile to attempt to conceal or ignore the gross disfigurement but it is essential to warn visitors who have not seen the condition, to be prepared and show no sign of repugnance. Sitting close to the patient, holding hands and talking as if there was no disfigurement at all are all helpful ways of desensitizing the patient. If it is possible to do it discreetly mirrors should be removed.

Physiology of dying

Some people assert that the process of dying begins with birth, but a more appropriate starting point is from the time when active efforts to cure the patient's illness have ceased and the doctor has decided as a result of clinical examination that the advent of death is not far away and that continuing care of the patient is concerned entirely with relieving distressing symptoms and ensuring that the remaining few days, weeks or months of the patient's life are comfortable.

The five vital systems of the body — the cardiovascular, pulmonary, gastro-intestinal, renal and central nervous systems have complex, mutually supportive interactions and if one system breaks down there is a knock-on effect on the other systems. As the deficiencies multiply a constantly changing kaleidoscope of symptoms develops. We know we cannot cure the patient and our concern is therefore to ensure by palliative care that none of these symptoms causes distress.

Causes of death

Once a patient has entered the terminal phase it must be accepted that sudden death is always a possibility and the relatives should be forewarned accordingly and at the same time given a full but simplified explanation of the patient's illness.

There may be a sudden internal or external haemorrhage due to tumour, erosion of a major blood vessel, a massive embolus affecting the lungs or brain, or a massive heart failure or acute pulmonary oedema.

It is more usual for the patient to move gradually towards the closing stages of life by progressive dysfunction of one or more of the major systems.

The cardiovascular system

Abnormalities within the heart itself, e.g. coronary disease may cause arrhythmias. There may be diminution of circulatory volume as in shock or haemorrhage. A breakdown of the other systems will also affect heart action, e.g. electrolytic disturbances or severe anaemia. The resultant defective pumping action of the heart in turn leads to hypoxia elsewhere.

Major resuscitative procedures are irrelevant for the heart failure supervening in terminal illness. It suffices to concentrate on controlling whatever symptoms arise which are distressing to the patient.

The pulmonary system

Defective oxygenation from pulmonary dysfunction may arise from: infection; tumour infiltration; bronchospasm or asthma; oedema; effusion; pneumothorax or infarct.

Specific symptomatic treatment should provide considerable relief from any distress occasioned by these conditions, but there remains a probability of the development of cerebral hypoxia. A common cause of death is infection leading to pneumonia.

The gastrointestinal and renal systems

Obstructions, infections, tumour infiltration and liver or renal failure may cause various toxic and electrolytic disturbances affecting heart and brain function. Uraemia, in particular, is common.

The central nervous system

It is on the activity of the nervous system that the integrity of the personality of the individual depends. The brain and spinal cord (being enclosed in a rigid bony structure) are particularly vulnerable to any condition causing increased pressure or occupying extra space. The factors that can damage the central nervous system are: infections, e.g. meningitis, encephalitis, brain abscess; blood vessel disruption or obstruction, e.g. thrombosis, haemorrhage, emboli; toxic and metabolic disorders, e.g. from renal or liver failure or extraneous poisons such as drugs; malignant tumours − primary or metastatic, and hypoxia due to circulatory or pulmonary failure. Hypoxia and defective blood circulation in the brain lead to the accumulation of toxic metabolites such as lactic acid. This is a major cause of brain death as this process initiates swelling which raises intracranial pressure and further reduces the circulation and oxygen supply.

The signs of central nervous system dysfunction are, in progression: confusion and disorientation; lethargy and apathy; stupor; semi-coma and coma. The deterioration is usually uneven and there are often marked fluctuations from one state to another.

Postural effects correlating with the brain damage may take the form of various types of paralysis, e.g. hemiparesis or spasticity of a limb or limbs.

Decorticate posture occurs in lethargy and stupor. Stimulation of the patient causes lower limb extension with toe pointing and upper limb flexion.

Decerebrate posture is associated with deeper unconsciousness − legs and arms extended and the palms are turned outwards.

In semi-coma the electroencephalogram changes in response to sensory stimulation. In what is called deep coma, there is no response to sensory stimuli but cortical rhythms persist in a relatively stable pattern. In terminal coma which is often seen in the final hour before respiration ceases, the cortical rhythm gradually melts into an isoelectric state which, however, is still not necessarily irreversible.

As brain hypoxia worsens the pupils dilate and eventually become unresponsive to light. The blood pressure falls and the pulse becomes rapid, feeble and irregular. Occasionally convulsive seizures may occur. Cheyne-Stokes breathing is very common with cerebral hypoxia and the rapid breathing is interrupted by periods of apnoea which become more and more prolonged.

Approaching death

No patient at this stage should ever be left alone. Someone sitting quietly holding the patient's hand will give great comfort and support. This is a time when family or friends are usually in constant watchful attendance. They should be kept fully informed about what is happening; for instance changing patterns of breathing and the nature and purpose of any treatment being given. The anguish of their grief will need constant support throughout this period, especially in the immediate aftermath of death.

Restlessness at this stage may be due to withdrawal reactions of the patient's medication when opiates have been suddenly discontinued. If the patient cannot take the medication orally it should be given by injection although a slightly reduced dose may suffice.

Faecal impaction should not have been allowed to develop but it may be a cause of much discomfort. Urinary retention is a common cause of restlessness and may easily be overlooked − catheterization will be necessary. Lying in an awkward position or on a pressure sore will obviously cause discomfort. Extreme dryness of the mouth and/or eyes is also uncomfortable. Moisturizing with methylcellulose applications is very soothing.

Noisy breathing (the death rattle) is due to secretions in the trachea and larynx which the patient is unable to cough up. If copious, suction will help and the patient should be placed well onto one side so that the secretions can drain away. An injection of hyoscine 0.4 mg may also be helpful or if there is pulmonary oedema, frusemide may be necessary.

If the patient continues to be restless, useful agents to help relaxation are Veractil (methotrimeprazine) 25 mg, Largactil (chlorpromazine) 50 mg or Ativan (lorazepam) 2 mg to 4 mg.

The restless legs syndrome in uraemia (also occurs in patients on renal dialysis) is thought to be due to disturbed function of brain stem reticular formation. It does not respond to any benzodiazepine except Rivotril (clonazepam) 0.5 mg bd or tds rising gradually to 2 mg tds if necessary, orally or intramuscularly.

Signs of death

These are absence of pulse and respiration and confirmed by absence of auscultatory sounds over the heart and trachea for at least five minutes. The pupils are fixed and dilated, and the fundi oculi show fragmentation of blood in the retinal veins.

Criteria for diagnosis of brain-stem death

Total loss of brain-stem function occurs when there are no spontaneous movements; no abnormal postures, i.e. no decorticate posturing, no decerebrate posturing; no epileptic jerking (these movements arise in the cortex and are routed through the brain-stem); no spontaneous respiration; no brain-stem reflexes i.e. no pupillary response to light, absent corneal reflex and no vestibulo-ocular reflexes. Any deviation of the eyes (or even of one eye) in response to irrigation of the tympanic membrane with ice-cold water implies live cells in the brain-stem; no facial movement in response to trigeminal input (firm supraorbital pressure); no oculo-cephalic reflexes (the presence of 'doll's head' eye movements implies live cells in the brain-stem); no gag reflex or reflex response to bronchial stimulation by suction catheter passed down the trachea.

All brain stem reflexes must be absent before brain-stem death can be diagnosed.

Rigor mortis is a contraction of muscle, so firm as to immobilize the joints, generally appearing in two to four hours after death, attaining its full intensity within forty-eight hours, and disappearing within another forty-eight hours. It begins in the jaw spreading downwards to involve the whole body and it disappears in the reverse direction. The time development is shortened in a warm atmosphere and when death occurs at a time of marked muscular activity. Reduction in adenosine triphosphate (ATP) is the chemical event that precipitates rigor mortis.

Postmortem decomposition

Decomposition of the body causes two main changes, discoloration and postmortem softening. Discoloration (hypostasis) starts immediately but is perceptible in two to three hours and fully established in eight to twelve hours. It is due to blood pigments and their derivatives. The red blood cells are haemolyzed after death, and the haemoglobin stains the vessel walls and the surrounding tissues. With the onset of putrefaction, sulphurated hydrogen is formed in the intestinal canal and combines with the iron of the breaking-down haemoglobin to form black sulphide of iron which stains the tissues green and black. The colour is first seen in the skin of the abdominal wall and on the surface of the abdominal organs.

Postmortem softening is due to the action of ferments: partly autolytic ferments in the tissues and partly the proteolytic ferments of the saprophytic bacteria causing putrefaction. The process is similar to that which occurs in moist gangrene. As a result of this fermentation the tissues are first softened and finally liquefied.

Transplants

Patients occasionally express a wish to donate their bodies for medical research. They should be asked to put this in writing, or if that is impossible to make their wishes known verbally before two witnesses, and this should then be documented in the case notes.

H.M. Inspector of Anatomy should be contacted. Pathological details will be required and if these prove acceptable instructions will be given as to the procedure when the patient dies.

Organs are not usually accepted from patients who have disseminated malignant disease.

Major transplants are usually obtained from young healthy people who have died from trauma.

Kidneys for transplant are much sought after. Contact the nearest Renal Unit before the patient dies if the patient has agreed or has signed a donor card.

Corneal transplants are very useful but they are only taken from patients free from eye disease and under 70 years of age. The eyes need to be removed within 36 hours. Ideally the local Eye Hospital should be alerted before the patient dies. Corneal transplants are acceptable in patients with malignant disease provided that the eyes have not been involved in the disease process.

Appendix 1

St. Joseph's Hospice
Advanced cancer admissions in a typical year

	Male	Female	Total
Beds available	30	30	60
Patients treated	415	425	840
Discharged	48	65	113
Died at St. Joseph's	367	360	727
Average Age	71	73	
Average length of stay	20 days	21 days	

Note 1   Not included in the above are six patients who proved to have either no cancer at all or who had cancer in such an early stage that it was amenable to treatment. Some of these cases could not be discharged for social reasons and have become long-stay patients

Note 2   CRITERIA FOR ADMISSION OF PATIENTS WITH ADVANCED CANCER

      1   The diagnosis of cancer has been confirmed

      2   The patient's condition has progressed beyond the stage when curative treatment is appropriate

      3   The prognosis, in so far as it can be established, is not more than six months

      4   Patients in the pre-terminal stage of cancer may also be admitted for some specific purpose − usually for control of a distressing symptom, e.g. pain or vomiting

If a doctor decides that a patient may eventually be a candidate for admission, early application is advised. This is preferable to waiting until the condition has reached the stage when emergency admission is required

The Medical Director is only too pleased to discuss with the patient's doctor any problem concerning admission and/or treatment of a patient suffering from advanced cancer

Note 3   Four beds are reserved for patients with motor neurone disease, either for respite care or for permanent admission

22 patients were treated during the year. 18 patients died

St. Joseph's Hospice.
Types of cancer in a typical year

	Male	Female	% of total (M + F)
Biliary tract	3	2	
Bladder	19	10	3.7
Brain	13	10	3.0
Breast	–	98	12.5
Caecum	3	6	
Colon	26	26	6.7
Kidney	3	7	
Larynx	4	3	
Leukaemia	2	1	
Liver	1	1	
Lung	124	49	22.2
Lymphoma	2	3	
Malignant melanoma	4	3	
Maxilla	–	1	
Mesothelioma	4	1	
Metastatic (Primary unidentified)	28	26	7.0
Middle ear	1	–	
Mouth	3	1	
Myeloma	3	1	
Nasopharynx	1	2	
Oesophagus	16	6	2.8
Ovary	–	19	
Pancreas	9	22	4.0
Prostate	36	–	4.6
Rectum	16	15	4.0
Sarcoma (chondro)	–	1	
Skin	4	3	
Stomach	37	16	6.8
Tonsil	1	–	
Thyroid	–	1	
Uterus – body	–	3	
Uterus – cervix	–	11	
Vulva	–	3	

Appendix 2

List of useful addresses:

Age Concern England
Bernard Sunley House
60 Pitcairn Road
Mitcham
Surrey
CR4 3LL

Age Concern Wales
Fourth floor
1 Cathedral Road
Cardiff
CF1 9S

Alzheimer's Disease Society
158–160 Balham High Road
London
SW12 9BN

Tel: 01 675 6557

BACUP
121–123 Charterhouse Street
London
EC1M 6AA

Tel: 01 608 1661

**Breast Care and Mastectomy
Association**
26 Harrison Street
Kings Cross
London
WC1 8JG

Tel: 01 837 0908

British Diabetic Association
10 Queen Anne Street
London
W1M 0BD

Tel: 01 323 1531

The British Epilepsy Association
Crowthorne House
Bigshotte
New Wokingham Road
Wokingham
Berkshire
RG11 3AY

Tel: 0344 3122

Cancer Relief MacMillan Fund
Anchor House
15/19 Britten Street
London
SW3 3TY

Tel: 01 351 7811

Child Poverty Action Group
1–5 Bath Street
London
EC1V 9PY

Colostomy Welfare Group
38–39 Eccleston Square
London
SW1V 1PB

Tel: 01 828 5175

The Compassionate Friends
(A self-help organisation of bereaved
parents)
6 Denmark Street
Bristol
BS1 5DQ

Tel: 0272 292778

CRUSE
126 Sheen Road
Richmond
Surrey
TW9 1UR

Tel: 01 940 4818

Disabled Living Foundation
380 Harrow Road
London
W9 2HU

Tel: 01 289 6111

Help the Aged
St James's Walk
London
EC1R 0BE

Help the Hospices
General Office
Tavistock Square
London
WC1H 9JP

Tel: 01 388 7807

The Leukaemia Society
45 Craigmoor Avenue
Bournemouth
Dorset

Tel: 0202 3749

Lisa Sainsbury Foundation
8 – 10 Crown Hill
Croydon
Surrey
CRO 1RY

Tel: 01 686 8808

Marie Curie Memorial Foundation
28 Belgrave Square
London
SW1X 8QG

Tel: 01 235 3325

Motor Neurone Disease Society
61 Derngate
Northampton
NN1 1UE

Tel: 0604 250505

The Multiple Sclerosis Society
286 Munster Road
London
SW6 6AP

Tel: 01 381 4022

**National Association of Laryngectomy
Clubs and Associates**
38 – 39 Eccleston Square
London

Tel: 01 834 2857

The National Association of Widows
1st floor
Neville House
14 Waterloo Street
Birmingham
B2 5TX

One Parent Families
255 Kentish Town Road
London
NW5 2LX

St. Christopher's Hospice
51 Lawrie Park Road
Sydenham
London
SE26 6DZ

Tel: 01 778 9252

St. Joseph's Hospice
Mare Street
Hackney
London
E8 4SA

Tel: 01 985 0861

Sue Ryder Home
Cavendish
Suffolk

Tel: 0787 280252

**The Royal National Institute for
the Blind**
224 – 228 Great Portland Street
London
W1N 6AA

Tel: 01 388 1266

The Royal National Institute for the Deaf
105 Gower Street
London
WC1E 6AH
Tel: 01 387 8033

Urinary Conduit Association
36 York Road
Deston
Manchester
Tel: 061 336 8818

The Samaritans
see local telephone book under 'S'

D49 leaflet *What to do after a death*, and other health and social security leaflets can be obtained from:

> DHSS Leaflets Unit,
> PO Box 21
> Stanmore
> HA7 1AY

Appendix 3

Corticosteroids in Terminal Cancer

Non-specific uses	Specific uses
1. To improve appetite	1. Hypercalcaemia
2. To enhance sense of well-being	2. Carcinomatous neuromyopathy
3. To improve strength	3. Incipient paraplegia
	4. Superior vena caval obstruction
Co-analgesic	5. Airways obstruction
	6. Haemoptysis
1. Raised intra-cranial pressure*	7. Leucoerythroblastic anaemia
2. Nerve compression	8. Malignant effusion*
3. Hepatomegaly	9. Discharge from rectal tumour**
4. Head and neck tumour*	10. To minimize radiation induced reactive oedema
5. Intra-pelvic tumour	
6. Abdominal tumour	11. To minimize the toxic effect of radiation or chemotherapy
7. Retroperitoneal tumour	
8. Lymphoedema*	12. As an adjunct to chemotherapy
9. Bone tumours	

* May benefit by concurrent use of a diuretic
** Given rectally (Predsol enema or suppository)

(a) Administer corticosteroids in form of prednisolone E.C. or dexamethasone and begin with large doses, if necessary by injection, to obtain a rapid response. Gradually reduce dose later as appropriate. Ranitidine 150 mg bd may be given concurrently to prevent gastric irritation.

(b) If corticosteroids are withdrawn from a patient who has been taking them for more than a week, this should be done gradually. A useful way to do this is to give one slow-release injection, e.g. Depo-Medrone 2 ml im.

Appendix 4

THE GRASEBY SYRINGE DRIVER

Requirements

1. Prescription from doctor
2. Syringe driver
3. Battery
4. 10 ml Monoject Syringe
5. Butterfly cannula and attached tubing [Vygen 246.100 Infusion Set]
6. Transparent dressing
7. i.e. Tegaderm, OpSite or Blenderm tape
8. Antiseptic swab

SETTING UP THE SYRINGE DRIVER

1. Full explanation of its purpose and how it works to patients and carers
2. Draw up medication and sterile water to a volume of 10 ml
3. Connect butterfly needle and tubing to syringe. If this is a new infusion prime tubing and needle with solution [approximately 0.5 ml]
4. Insert battery and keep spare battery available
5. Press start/test button. Machine will produce a soft whirring and indicator light will flash on/off
6. Check rate is set correctly on front of syringe driver. [Usually set to deliver contents of syringe in 25 hours. 10 ml syringe measures 50 mm therefore rate set on 2 mm per hour]
7. Fit syringe with infusion tubing and needle attached to syringe driver. Place flange of syringe in slot provided and secure with rubber strap. Extra tape may be used to secure syringe to pump
8. Fit plunger. Press white release button, then slide plunger assembly until it presses against syringe plunger. Pump is now ready for use

INSERTING THE CANNULA

1. Choose a site for the butterfly needle. The most useful sites are the upper chest, outer aspect of upper arm, abdomen and thighs [never in an oedematous area]

2. Insert the needle at 45 degrees subcutaneously
3. Cover butterfly with transparent dressing. Anchor small circle of tubing to prevent 'pulling' on butterfly
4. Place clear plastic case into the holster and insert the pump into the case

Notes

Site should be checked daily and changed if area is inflamed, painful or lumpy

Start/test button may be used to deliver small extra dose, e.g. prior to changing a painful dressing

Light stops flashing when battery is low; pump will continue to operate for 24 hours after this. Battery lasts approximately six weeks

Appendix 5

SOCIAL HISTORY

NAME: SEX: DATE OF ADMISSION:

ADDRESS: DATE OF BIRTH: AGE:

     PLACE OF BIRTH:

ACCOMMODATION: MARITAL STATUS:

OCCUPATION: RELIGION:
(Or previous occupation)

FAMILY Note sex and approx. age Note carers (C) Note bereavement risk (B)	PARENTS	SIBLINGS	SPOUSE	CHILDREN

OTHER CARING FRIENDS

NEXT OF KIN

NAME: RELATIONSHIP:

ADDRESS: TEL: DAY

     NIGHT

OTHER CONTACT

NAME: RELATIONSHIP:

ADDRESS: TEL: DAY

     NIGHT

GP

NAME: HOSPITAL

ADDRESS: CONSULTANT:

TEL:

MEDICAL HISTORY

NAME: AGE: WARD:

ADMITTED FROM: ADMITTING DR:

REASON(S)   DATE:

DIAGNOSIS 1

  2 DEPOSITS

OTHER ILLNESSES

PRESENT ILLNESS

WHEN FIRST ILL

WHEN DIAGNOSED:

SURGERY:

HORMONE/CHEMOTHERAPY

RADIOTHERAPY

RECENT INVESTIGATIONS

CURRENT SYMPTOMS

		MEDICATION PRIOR TO ADMISSION
ANOREXIA	BOWELS	
DYSPHAGIA	MICT	
NAUSEA	INCONTINENCE	
VOMITING	DISCHARGE	
WEIGHT		

DYSPNOEA	BLEEDING
– AT REST	FISTULA
– ON EXERTION	MENTAL STATE
COUGH	
MOBILITY	SLEEP

INSIGHT   PATIENT'S EXPECTATIONS AND FEELINGS

DIAGNOSIS

PROGNOSIS   RELATIVES' EXPECTATIONS AND FEELINGS

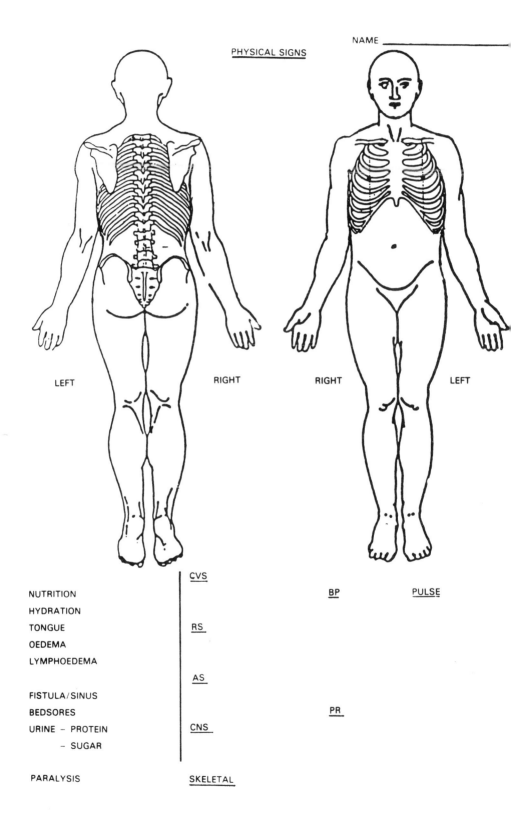

PHYSICAL SIGNS

NAME _____

LEFT　　　　　RIGHT　　　　　RIGHT　　　　　LEFT

	CVS	
NUTRITION		BP　　　PULSE
HYDRATION		
TONGUE	RS	
OEDEMA		
LYMPHOEDEMA		
	AS	
FISTULA/SINUS		
BEDSORES		PR
URINE – PROTEIN	CNS	
– SUGAR		
PARALYSIS	SKELETAL	

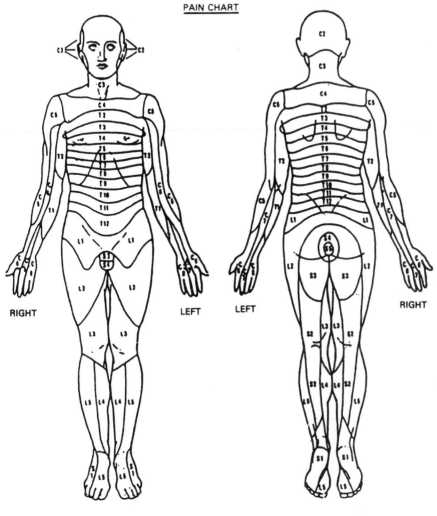

PAIN CHART

RIGHT   LEFT   LEFT   RIGHT

SEVERITY (MILD (1) — (4) SEVERE)   CAUSE

PAIN A

PAIN B

PAIN C

PROBLEMS   TREATMENT

Index